Wound Care Nursing

For Elsevier:

Associate Editor: Dinah Thom
Project Development Manager: Mairi McCubbin
Project Manager: Caroline Horton
Design direction: Judith Wright
Illustrations Manager: Bruce Hogarth

Wound Care Nursing

A patient-centred approach

SECOND EDITION

Sue Bale BA PhD PGDip DipN RGN NDN RMV FRCN

Associate Director of Nursing, Gwent Healthcare NHS Trust, South Wales, UK

Vanessa Jones MSc PGCE RGN NDN RCNT

Senior Lecturer/Education Director, Wound Healing Research Unit, Department of Surgery, Cardiff University, Cardiff, UK

Foreword by
Christine Moffatt MA PhD RGN DN
Professor of Nursing, Faculty of Health and Human Sciences, Thames Valley University, London, UK

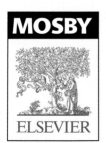

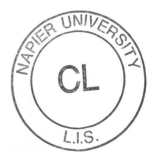

EDINBURGH LONDON NEW YORK OXFORD PHILADELPHIA ST LOUIS SYDNEY TORONTO 2006

MOSBY
ELSEVIER

© 1997 Baillière Tindall
© Harcourt Publishers Limited 2000
© 2006, Elsevier Limited. All rights reserved.

First edition 1997
Second edition 2006

ISBN 0 7234 3344 5

British Library Cataloguing in Publication Data
A catalogue record for this book is available from the British Library

Library of Congress Cataloging in Publication Data
A catalog record for this book is available from the Library of Congress

Notice
Knowledge and best practice in this field are constantly changing. As new research and experience broaden our knowledge, changes in practice, treatment and drug therapy may become necessary or appropriate. Readers are advised to check the most current information provided (i) on procedures featured or (ii) by the manufacturer of each product to be administered, to verify the recommended dose or formula, the method and duration of administration, and contraindications. It is the responsibility of the practitioner, relying on their own experience and knowledge of the patient, to make diagnoses, to determine dosages and the best treatment for each individual patient, and to take all appropriate safety precautions. To the fullest extent of the law, neither the Publisher nor the Authors assumes any liability for any injury and/or damage to persons or property arising out or related to any use of the material contained in this book.

The Publisher

Printed in China

CONTENTS

FOREWORD

The second edition of this book will be widely welcomed by specialist and generalist nurses caring for patients with wounds in all health-care settings in the United Kingdom as well as other English speaking parts of the world.

This is a highly readable book written by two eminent nurses in the field of wound care, who together have made a major contribution to the profile and professionalism of nursing. It is a delight to see the integration of nursing theory throughout this book and the way in which the authors use different nursing models to address the complex needs of individual patients. The consideration of the different needs of different age groups is also particularly unique and will widen its appeal to those working in specialist settings. The inclusion of case studies drawn from the authors' extensive clinical experience will allow nurses to apply the evidence based recommendations to the care of their patients.

If every nurse involved in wound care were to have access to this book and apply the sound principles within it, there would be an immediate improvement in care, with improved healing and cost effectiveness and a reduction in patient suffering. I highly recommend this book to all those seeking to improve patient care.

Christine Moffatt

PREFACE

Wounds are a common clinical problem, cared for in most, if not all, clinical settings including hospital wards and the community. As we experience change towards an increasingly elderly population with people living longer, the number of people with chronic wounds is set to rise. Chronic wounds, including pressure, leg and diabetic foot ulcers, adversely affect patients' lives as they experience lengthy healing times, pain, psychological distress and delays in returning to normal activity. Although wound management has developed into a speciality that is broadly multi-professional, it is one where nurses continue to provide much of the delivery of care.

With clinical governance comes a growing awareness of the risks related to failing to deliver high standards of wound care as well as the benefits derived from providing an excellent service to patients. In the past the delivery of nursing care has been subjected to criticism because of its frequent adherence to ritualistic practices, and wound care has been particularly targeted for such criticism. Nursing has embraced the drive towards evidence-based practice and wound management is no exception to this. There are many societies and associations, journals, web sites, books and conferences dedicated solely to the problems of managing patients with wounds. Many of the books currently available are for the post-registered nurse or practitioner who has some experience in this field and they assume a corresponding level of knowledge .

This book aims to be different by linking the holistic approach that is so important in nursing with nursing theory. For many nurses in clinical practice, nursing theory is unfamiliar, with limited relevance to their daily practice. The new approach taken in the first edition continues in this edition. We use the nursing process and nursing models to help the reader see how *theory can be applied to practice*. This book is designed to meet the needs of those new to wound care nursing. By developing the skills of assessment, planning and management and evaluation of care, the reader can focus on patients and their wound-related problems. We hope that this approach helps the student nurse and non-specialist nurses in hospital and the community to place wound care in the context of nursing generally. Here, wound care becomes integrated into and part of the evaluation of patient care as a whole as well as in relation to local wound care.

Although there is increasing activity in scientific research by scientists, our understanding of the science of wound healing is limited. While this work continues nurses must utilize the research evidence generated so far and deliver care based on the best evidence that is available. To this end the material contained in this book is based on research evidence and is referenced extensively. Suggested further reading is provided for those readers who wish to pursue topics of interest in more depth.

The life-cycle chapters provide case study material that brings each chapter to life by demonstrating how the theory is applied in practice. Each chapter contains examples of care plans where readers have the opportunity to work through and formulate care plans of their own, using a model of their own choosing. This interactive element of the book is designed to encourage the reader to take an analytical approach, apply knowledge and develop problem-solving skills.

This book can also be used by experienced wound care practitioners to enhance practice and help them determine their responsibilities of preceptorship with students and less experienced colleagues. Nurses working and studying in the community will find that a significant proportion of the patient cases are community based, thus reflecting the setting in which most patients are cared for. However, the majority of information is relevant to wound care regardless of the health-care setting.

The book is divided into three sections, reflecting the stages of the nursing process:

Section 1. This section presents assessment and planning of care, providing the theoretical knowledge required for the reader to proceed to the next section.

Section 2. This section illustrates how this theoretical knowledge can be transferred into practice. A life-cycle approach is taken where each chapter covers a different age group from birth to old age. It begins with babies and young children, moves through the teenage years to young adulthood and middle age, and concludes with two chapters devoted to the older group. Each stage of the life cycle provides the reader with an insight into the range and variety of wound healing problems that typically affect that age group, utilizing nursing models that are appropriate to those groups. Real-life patient cases help the reader to draw together assessment and planning of care with expected outcomes.

Section 3. This final section discusses evaluation of care, providing a structured framework for this process.

We hope that by reading this book and working through the Practice Points provided, nurses will be able to relate each chapter to their own experience, so broadening their knowledge base and enhancing their status as professionals.

Sue Bale
Vanessa Jones

Please note that all names used in the patient case studies are fictitious.
Words appearing emboldened in the text are explained in the Glossary.

ACKNOWLEDGEMENTS

All clinical pictures, other than those acknowledged individually in the accompanying captions, were kindly supplied by Professor K G Harding, Wound Healing Research Unit, Cardiff University.

Assessment and Planning

CHAPTER 1

Assessing the normal and abnormal

Case study 1.1

Adenocarcinoma of the rectum

Mr David Simons, a 52-year-old man, had previously been admitted to hospital with a history of rectal bleeding, intermittent diarrhoea and lower abdominal colic.

He was diagnosed as having an invasive adenocarcinoma of the rectum and treated with radiotherapy and chemotherapy. Surgery was not planned at that stage as he was still opening his bowels without difficulty and it was decided to reassess the patient after treatment.

Prior to the initial consultation David had lost 45 kg in weight and had separated from his wife, who lived with their eight children in a two-bedroomed flat, while he lived in a YMCA hostel.

Following treatment he was due to return some weeks later with a view to surgery for a defunctioning colostomy but was admitted in the interim period with a one-week history of a swollen, painful right leg.

David was cachetic, with pyrexia (37.5°C); blood tests revealed a haemoglobin level of 7.9 g/dl and a serum albumin concentration of 18 g/l. His leg was swollen from hip to foot, especially over the lateral aspect of his thigh, where there was also evidence of surgical emphysema.

Emergency surgery revealed that the colon had perforated owing to the advancing tumour and the colonic contents had caused surgical emphysema in the tissue of the right leg. Infection had spread rapidly, causing necrotizing fasciitis and therefore gross destruction of the tissue and muscle of the pelvis, hip and thigh region.

David was taken to theatre three times over the following five days for excision and debridement of the **necrotic tissue** and formation of a colostomy. The wounds that resulted from this surgical intervention (Figure 1.1) were:

- large cavity down to muscle fascia and penetrating into the pelvic cavity on the lateral aspect of the hip, drained with a size 36 sump drain tube
- cavity on the medial aspect of the thigh
- 10×6 cm cavity on the lateral calf
- 3×2 cm cavity on the dorsum of the foot.

Thought unlikely to survive the initial surgery, he did survive, and postoperatively David became depressed and withdrawn, was in a great deal of pain, especially at dressing changes and was unable to tolerate any substantial diet.

INTRODUCTION

The problems described in Case study 1.1 are not typical of those facing nurses in their day-to-day work. However, Mr Simon's case is an excellent example of a complex clinical situation where many factors that can complicate the normal process of healing are present. This illustrates the importance of the nurse's role in being able to assess clinical situations. The effective management of patients with wounds and wound problems depends upon the nurse's ability to recognize normality and abnormality in healing by taking a systematic, logical, holistic approach. This organized approach consists of assessment of the individual, the wound and the environment (Figure 1.2).

Figure 1.1
David Simons following
emergency surgery.

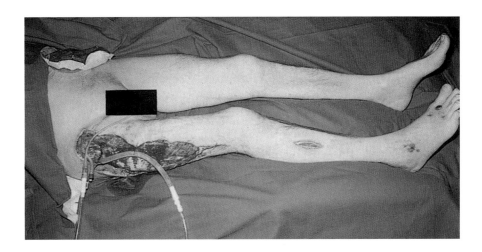

Figure 1.2
A holistic approach to
wound assessment.

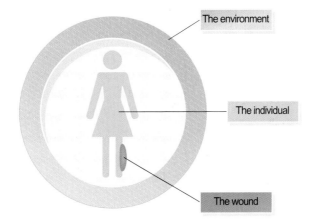

The environment

The individual

The wound

**ASSESSMENT OF
THE INDIVIDUAL**

Assessment of the overall health of the individual will highlight factors that
may impair the normal healing process, though before an understanding of
these factors can be appreciated it is essential that the nurse is knowledgeable
about the normal healing process.

**Normal wound
healing**

Wound healing is a complex chain of events that can be divided into its four
constituent phases, **haemostasis, inflammation, proliferation** and **maturation** (Figure 1.3), all of which overlap.

It should be remembered that these processes take place concurrently and
do not always follow one another in an orderly sequence.

Haemostasis

Following cutaneous injury to blood vessels and endothelial cells, blood
extravasation into the wound defect exposes the blood to various components
of the extracellular matrix (ECM) (Witte & Barbul 1997). Platelets aggregate
and degranulate, resulting in clot formation and **haemostasis**. Haemostasis is
the arrest of haemorrhage at the site of blood vessel damage and is essential as
it preserves the integrity of the closed and high-pressure circulatory system in

Figure 1.3
The wound healing process. Although for convenience the wound healing process is considered here in four phases, it is important to remember that healing is a dynamic, ongoing process. It begins at day 0 with initial wounding but can continue for several years.

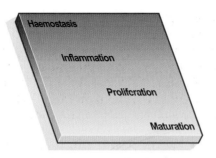

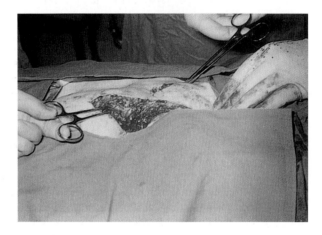

Figure 1.4
Haemostasis.

order to limit blood loss (Figure 1.4). A fibrinous clot forms during coagulation. This acts as a preliminary matrix within the wound space into which cells can migrate. A short period of vasoconstriction occurs owing to the release of chemical mediators such as histamine, serotonin and adenosine triphosphate (ATP). Most of these mediators act as chemoattractants to circulating **leucocytes**, bringing them to the injured area.

Following initial vasoconstriction, the inflammatory process begins with the release of prostaglandins and activated complement proteins, causing widespread vasodilation and inflammation (Iocono et al 1998).

Inflammatory phase
As the fibrin clot is degraded, the capillaries dilate and become permeable, thus allowing plasma to leak into the surrounding tissue, producing inflammatory exudate. This activates the complement system, composed of a series of interacting, soluble proteins found in serum and extracellular fluid that induce lysis and destruction of target cells, such as bacteria. Cytokines and some proteolytic fragments that are chemoattractive are also found in the wound space (Steed 1997). Their abundance and accumulation at the site of wounding initiate a massive influx of other cells.

The two main inflammatory cells are neutrophils and macrophages (Martin 1997). Neutrophils appear in a wound shortly after injury and reach their peak number within 24–48 hours. Their main function is to destroy bacteria by the process of phagocytosis. Neutrophils have a very short lifespan and their numbers reduce rapidly after three days in the absence of infection. Monocytes undergo a phenotypic change to become activated **macrophages,** which produce growth factors that start, accelerate or modify the healing process. Tissue macrophages, like neutrophils, destroy bacteria and debris through phagocytosis. The macrophage is also a rich source of biological regulators, including cytokines and growth factors, bio-active lipid products and proteolytic enzymes, which are also essential for the normal healing process (Slavin1999, Steed 1997)

The formation of new blood vessels occurs with the release of **angiogenic** growth factors which stimulate **endothelium** to divide and direct the growth of new blood vessels (Lingen & Nickoloff 2001).

Proliferative phase

The macrophages next recruit a new type of cell, the **fibroblast**, which produces a network of **collagen** surrounding the neovasculature of the wound. Fibroblasts also produce proteoglycans, a glue-like ground substance which fills the tissue space, coating and binding fibres together to give them greater flexibility and fibronectin, which forms the framework for tissue by holding collagen and cells together while attaching them to the ground substance.

The **proliferation** phase usually commences at about day three following injury and lasts for some weeks. This phase is characterized by the formation of granulation tissue in the wound space, this new tissue consisting of a matrix of fibrin, fibronectin, collagens, proteoglycans and glycosaminoglycans and other glycoproteins (Hart 2002). Fibroblasts move into the wound space and proliferate; their function during wound healing is to synthesize and deposit extracellular proteins, producing growth factors and angiogenic factors that regulate cell proliferation and angiogenesis (Stephens & Thomas 2002).

Collagen is the most abundant protein in animal tissue and accounts for 70–80% of the dry weight of the dermis (Wysocki 2000). Mainly made by fibroblasts, there are at least 19 genetically distinct collagens currently identified. Collagen synthesis and degradation are finely balanced (Slavin 1999). Elastin is a protein that provides wounds with elasticity and resilience (Wysocki 2000). Elastin fibres form coils that enable it to stretch and return to its former shape, much like metallic coils. Because of these properties, elastin helps to maintain tissue shape.

The role of exudate Wound exudate is initially produced in the inflammatory phase of healing (Cutting 2004, White 2001), though it continues to be produced throughout the healing phase until complete **epithelialization** has been achieved. Exudate has a high protein content and contains essential nutrients as well as providing a moist environment (Cutting 2004). These include plasma proteins, growth factors, proteolytic enzmes, glucose, lactic acid, white blood cells, macrophages, fibrin and platelets (Cutting 2004).

Measuring and describing levels of exudate production for the purposes of evaluating progress towards healing and recording wound symptoms is largely a subjective process. Bates-Jensen (1997) has developed a scale that can be used to chart exudate levels. The descriptors range from none to large (volume of exudate), where large is quantified as wound tissues bathed in fluid and drainage that involves 75% of the dressing.

Figure 1.5
Healthy granulation tissue on the wound bed of a pilonidal sinus excision (reproduced with kind permission from the *Journal of Wound Care*, London).

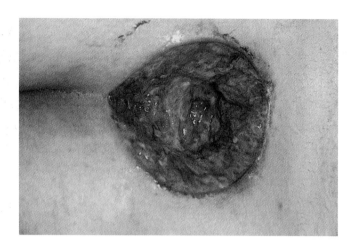

The formation of new connective tissue (granulation tissue) is dependent on angiogenesis with the resultant formation of new blood vessels in the wound (Figure 1.5). Initially the wound is hypoxic and lacking in nutrients but as capillary loops are formed, the environment becomes oxygenated (Lingen & Nickoloff 2001). Angiogenesis or formation of new vessels in the wound space is an integral and essential part of wound healing (Neal 2001). The major cell involved in angiogenesis is the vascular endothelial cell, which arises from the damaged end of vessels and capillaries. New vessels originate as capillaries, which sprout from existing small vessels at the wound edge. The endothelial cells from these vessels are detached from the vascular wall, degrade and penetrate (invade) the provisional matrix in the wound, thus forming a cone-shaped vascular bud or sprout. A sprout is then extended in length until it encounters another capillary and connects to form vascular loops and networks, allowing blood to circulate.

During proliferation, two other processes are taking place simultaneously – epithelialization and contraction. Epithelialization resurfaces the wound by regenerating epithelium. Where damage is extensive and involves deep dermal tissue loss, regeneration occurs from the wound margins. Where there is superficial skin loss, remnants of hair follicles will act as islands of regenerating epithelium. Migration across the wound surface continues until other epithelial cells are met. The migration then ceases, a complex process known as contact inhibition. Wound contraction decreases the size of the wound, a process largely due to the work of the **myofibroblast**. Myofibroblasts under the influence of inflammatory mediators reduce the surface area of the wound before cellular proliferation takes place. The myofibroblast is a differentiated fibroblast containing actin and myosin fibrils (Whitby 1995).

Once an open cavity has filled with new granulation tissue and epithelialization has occurred, the proliferative phase of healing stops.

Maturation phase
The final stage of healing begins roughly three weeks after injury and is a process of remodelling of the collagen fibres laid down during the proliferation phase (Figure 1.6).

Figure 1.6
A healed pilonidal sinus excision in the maturation phase.

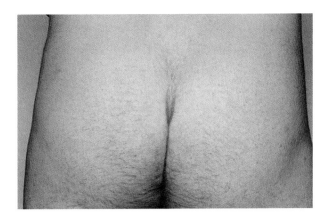

During the maturation phase, type III collagen, a soft gelatinous collagen, is gradually replaced with stronger, more highly organized collagen. Differentiation of collagen is a dynamic process and although it commences predominantly during maturation, it may continue indefinitely.

Collagen breakdown and production is a finely balanced process which, if impaired, can result in delayed or inadequate healing. Once established, the amount of collagen bed does not alter, just the type and formation within the wound. Type III collagen is removed by collagenases and synthesis of type I collagen occurs, laid down in a more orderly network, fashioned along the lines of tension.

The process of remodelling continues with the fibroblasts migrating from the wound site and there is rationalization of the numerous blood vessels, resulting in shrinking, thinning and paling of the scar.

Healing by primary intention

Healing by primary intention occurs following a clean surgical incision where the edges of the wound are closely approximated, thus eliminating dead space. There is minimal formation of granulation tissue and once the wound has healed, only a thin seam remains. All the above phases of wound healing occur but following the initial inflammatory response, wound contraction has a minor role and epithelium migrates over the **suture** line to restore tissue integrity (Cho & Hunt 2001).

Healing by secondary intention

Healing by secondary intention (Figure 1.7) occurs in wounds where there is a large tissue defect. The wound must heal by formation of granulation tissue and wound contraction, resulting in dense, fibrous scar tissue. Generally these wounds take longer to heal because of the large amounts of granulation tissue required. The proliferative and maturation phases are longer than in wounds healing by primary intention.

Healing by third intention

Where the presence of **infection** or a foreign body is suspected, a wound may be left open to commence healing by granulation until the presenting problem has been resolved. The wound edges are then approximated and healing by primary intention can proceed.

Figure 1.7
An axillary wound healing by secondary intention.

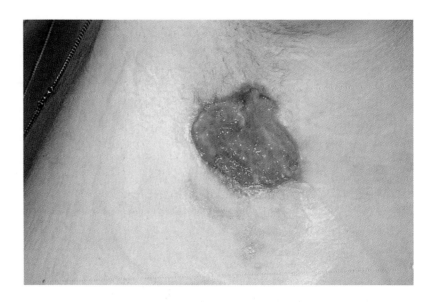

Abnormal wound healing

Unfortunately, failure or delay in achieving adequate healing is relatively common, especially for patients with chronic wounds. Abnormalities of wound healing are described below.

Dehiscence

Dehiscence occurs when the wound has failed to develop sufficient strength to withstand forces placed upon it. Good surgical technique should prevent complications such as wound dehiscence, which is often the result of a technical failure by the surgeon (Bale & Leaper 2000), by placing the sutures in areas associated with collagenolysis. Wound dehiscence usually occurs around 6–10 days postoperatively, although it can occur up to a month after surgery.

The patient often presents with pyrexia and wound discharge of serosanguineous fluid. The risk is always increased by localized wound infection, **haematoma** formation or excessive tension placed on the wound by coughing.

Incisional hernia

Incisional hernias (Figure 1.8) occur in up to 10% of abdominal wounds (Robson et al 1997) and can develop months or even years following surgery and represent failure of part of the scar to develop sufficient strength. They occur more often in infected wounds and in the obese. The risk factors include hypoxia, immunosuppressant treatments, metabolic disorders, obesity, previous abdominal surgery, previous incisional hernia and wound dehiscence (Robson et al 1997).

Malignant changes

Any long-standing ulcer may undergo malignant changes to form a squamous cell carcinoma. Although the precise mechanism is unknown, with such a rapid turnover of cells in any wound it is important that the practitioner should bear in mind the possibility of malignancy.

Figure 1.8
An incisional hernia.

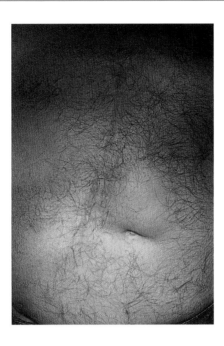

Table 1.1
Factors adversely affecting
the healing process

Intrinsic factors	Extrinsic factors
Age	Poor surgical technique
Disease processes/metabolic	Poor wound care
Psychological status	Malnutrition
Body image	Fluid balance Smoking Drug therapies Radiotherapy

Any wound that has an unusual appearance or fails to heal over a long period should be investigated. Rojas and Phillips (2001) recommend that as between 0.34% and 9% of leg ulcers are malignant, those patients who have failed to heal over an expected period should be routinely biopsied to exclude malignancy.

FACTORS AFFECTING WOUND HEALING

There are many factors that can adversely affect the normal healing process, including those that are intrinsic and those that are extrinsic. Some of these factors can be prevented or treated by careful assessment and some cannot.

Key factors adversely affecting wound healing are listed in Table 1.1. Assessment aims to identify these factors and, wherever possible, treat or prevent them. However, where this is not possible, factors known to affect healing should be documented and the possibility of delayed healing planned for.

Intrinsic factors

Age
In old age the dermis of skin gradually becomes thinner and the underlying structural support, collagen, is reported by Hunter (1995) to diminish at a rate

of 1% per annum. Skin loses elasticity as the fibroblasts responsible for elastin and collagen synthesis decline in number, elastic fibres thicken and the ability for elastic recoil is lost, so causing creases and wrinkles. At the same time the amount of subcutaneous fat lessens, so providing less of a cushion for underlying bone. Additionally, natural moisture from sebum secretion reduces in old age as these sweat glands become smaller, leading to increased dryness of the skin. Overall, the ageing process adversely affects skin quality, causing dry, thin inelastic skin that is susceptible to damage. With advancing age the metabolic processes – including the wound-healing process – begin to slow down, so prolonging the healing phase. Tensile wound strength is often affected owing to reduced collagen production and poor circulation associated with old age.

Disease

A whole range of disease processes that adversely affect metabolism are also likely to delay or prevent wound healing.

- Anaemia
- **Arteriosclerosis**
- Cancer
- Cardiovascular disorders
- Diabetes
- Immune disorders
- Inflammatory diseases
- Jaundice, liver failure
- Rheumatoid arthritis
- Uraemia.

In some vulnerable groups of patients, especially the elderly, several disease processes may be present in one individual at the same time.

Psychological factors

There is a close association between the psychological and physical well-being of individuals and psychological problems can have an adverse effect on the health of patients. Stress and anxiety in particular can affect the immune system (Waldrop & Doughty 2000). Stress has been shown to affect serum levels of corticosteroid, which impairs immune function (Keicolt-Glaser 1995). Animal and human laboratory studies have also demonstrated the effects of stress on the sympathetic nervous system, where vasoactive substances (for example, catecholamines) impair perfusion to the wound bed (Padgett et al 1998, Stotts & Wipke-Tevis 1997). Waldrop and Doughty recommend that wound assessment plans should take into account psychological factors that may delay healing and also address factors such as pain control, guided imagery, patient education and counselling.

Sleep disturbances are also linked with stress. Sleep is thought to be essential for healing and tissue repair. Sleep encourages anabolism and, as wound healing includes anabolic processes, it has been suggested that healing is promoted by rest and sleep. Dealey (1999) reviewed the literature regarding sleep and healing, reporting that growth hormone is secreted during sleep, which in turn stimulates protein synthesis and fibroblast and endothelial cell proliferation. She also discusses sleep disturbance during hospitalization, suggesting that with careful planning many of the factors that disturb sleep in hospital can be eliminated.

Body image

Body image has been defined as an individual's perception of their own appearance, which may be quite different from their actual physical appearance (Rodgers 1999). Body image can be adversely altered or affected by a change in physical appearance such as traumatic injury, surgery or burns (Bale & Morison 1997). Developing a chronic wound can also affect or change an individual's body image. Dramatic negative effects can occur especially when disfiguring surgery has been performed such as mastectomy, stoma formation or the amputation of a limb. The grieving process is associated with this negative alteration in body image (Dealey 1999); common problems include a sense of loss, anxiety and withdrawal from social relationships.

Extrinsic factors

Poor surgical technique

Specific situations which may impair healing include: inadequate closure of tissue layers, resulting in a dead space; inappropriate use of diathermy or drains; sutures inserted too tightly or too loosely; prolonged operating time and haematoma (Leaper & Harding 2000b). The most common of these problems is haematoma formation, caused by rough handling of tissues and by inappropriate use of diathermy or wound drains. This can lead to the presence of a dead space, encouraging wound infection as the haematoma is broken down. Kindlen and Morison (1997) describe complications from haematoma formation that include: increased tension on the healing wound; excess fibrosis or scar tissue; and, most commonly, the excellent medium provided for micro-organisms that increases the risk of infection and wound breakdown.

Poor wound care

Wound healing may be impeded by poor dressing technique or the inappropriate use of a dressing material or antiseptic solution. These problems can be avoided by careful assessment by a practitioner with a sound knowledge and understanding of the principles of managing patients with wounds.

Malnutrition

Malnutrition can result in delays in wound healing, resulting in weak, poor-quality scars. In reviewing the literature on malnutrition and healing, McLaren (1997) and Stotts (2000) describe two types of malnutrition that affect healing: protein-energy malnutrition (PEM) and nutrient deficiencies.

Protein-energy malnutrition (PEM) McLaren (1997) defines PEM as a change in body composition and physiology that results from an absolute or relative deficiency of energy and protein, which affects between 19% and 50% of hospitalized patients. She attributes PEM to several factors including a reduced intake of nutrients, reduced absorption and digestion of nutrients and increased metabolic use. McLaren (1997) estimates that although 70% of these patients are malnourished prior to admission, the remaining 30% develop PEM during their hospital stay, as a complication.

Box 1.1 Patients at risk of hospital-induced protein-energy malnutrition (from Dickerson 1995)

1. Emergency admission
2. All age groups but especially elderly individuals recently bereaved, socially isolated or with sensory or mental impairment
3. Malignancy, especially cancer of the gastrointestinal tract
4. Alimentary tract diseases
5. Dysphagia or anorexia

Dickerson (1995) identified a range of patients vulnerable to hospital-induced PEM (Box 1.1). Other research supports this. McWhirter and Pennington (1994) found that 200 out of 500 patients admitted to hospital were undernourished and just over 100 lost weight during their admission. Gray and Cooper (2001) and the European Pressure Ulcer Advisory Panel (EPUAP 2003) recommend that nutritional screening tools should be used to identify patients at risk of being malnourished and that food record charts are also useful in ensuring that patients receive optimal care. Malnutrition can affect wound healing in several ways.

- Poor wound healing, reduced tensile strength and increased wound dehiscence (Dickerson 1995, Stotts & Whitney 1990)
- Increased susceptibility to infections (Dickerson 1995)
- Susceptibility to the development of pressure ulcers (Dickerson 1995, Meaume et al 1994)
- Poor-quality scarring (Pinchcofsky-Devin 1994).

Specific requirements for individual patients vary and depend on their body weight. The EPUAP nutrition guidelines (EPUAP 2003) are based on a systematic review of the literature and recommend a minimum intake of 30–35 kcal per kg of body weight, with 1–1.5 g per kg per day protein and 1 ml per kcal per day of fluid intake. EPUAP (2003) recommends that health professionals should consider the quality of the food being offered, along with removing physical or social barriers to its consumption. It also suggests that nutritional supplements be considered when it is not possible to enhance the patient's own consumption of food and fluids.

Trace element deficiency Zinc is an essential cofactor for the enzymatic activity of 200 or more enzymes, including protein synthesis (McLaren 1992, Williams 2002) and zinc deficiency has long been known to impair wound healing (Gray & Cooper 2001). Patients who are zinc deficient have reduced rates of epithelialization, decreased wound strength and reduced collagen synthesis (Pinchcofsky-Devin 1994).

Copper is needed for the cross-linkage of collagen. Although rare, copper deficiency reduces the activity of an enzyme, lysyl oxidase, essential in collagen formation. Patients receiving long-term total parenteral nutrition and those with malabsorption syndrome are most at risk (McLaren 1992).

Collagen synthesis relies on *iron* as it is an essential cofactor for both lysyl and prolyl hydroxylase. In addition, anaemia may impair healing through reducing oxygen transportation (McLaren 1992).

Vitamin deficiency   *Vitamin C* is essential for the synthesis of collagen. It functions as a cofactor in the hydroxylation of proline to hydroxyproline (Pinchcofsky-Devin 1994). A deficiency in vitamin C results in impaired angiogenesis (Williams 2002), reduces tensile strength within wounds, impairs angiogenesis and increases capillary fragility (Gray & Cooper 2001, McLaren 1992).

Vitamin A enhances the early inflammatory response, whilst stimulating fibroblast proliferation and increasing tensile strength (Williams 2002). It may also be linked to limiting wound infections as it is important in the normal human defence mechanism. It is also involved in the cross-linking of collagen and the proliferation of epithelial cells (Gray & Cooper 2001). Supplements of vitamin A have been used to reverse the effects of corticosteroid treatments in patients, to improve wound healing (Pinchcofsky-Devin 1994).

Fluid balance

In addition to an adequate intake of food, fluids are also required. Around 2000–2500 ml of fluid are required daily for efficient metabolism.

Smoking

Smoking has an adverse effect on the general health of individuals throughout their lives. There is a high correlation between smoking, lung cancer and cardiovascular diseases. Tobacco smoke contains nicotine and carbon monoxide. There are, however, differences between cigarette smoke and pipe or cigar smoke as far as nicotine is concerned, cigarettes being more harmful to health (Siana et al 1992) with more nicotine being absorbed and peripheral blood flow being depressed by at least 50% for more than an hour after smoking just one cigarette. In animal models nicotine has been shown to inhibit epithelialization (Waldrop & Doughty 2000); human smokers have been shown to have postoperative problems with scarring (Siana et al 1989). On the other hand, no specific research has evaluated the influence of carbon monoxide on healing (Siana et al 1992). There is a plethora of research on the detrimental effects of carbon monoxide on blood vessels and blood components suggestive of a probable effect on wound healing (Table 1.2).

Drug therapies

Drugs that interfere with cell proliferation can have a severe effect on wound healing. These are predominantly cytotoxic drugs, especially vincristine.

Table 1.2
The main influence of nicotine and carbon monoxide on peripheral tissue in relation to wound healing (reproduced with kind permission from Siana et al 1992)

Tissue	Nicotine	Carbon monoxide	Total effect
Skin	Contraction	Dilation	Contraction
Muscles	Dilation		Dilation
Oxygen supply	Reduced blood flow	Reduced oxygen transport	Reduced oxygen tension in tissue
Platelets	Increased aggregation	Increased aggregation	Formation of thrombi
Fibrin	Increased plasma concentration		No proven effect

Figure 1.9
Hypertrophic scarring (reproduced with kind permission from Dr C Lawrence, Wound Healing Research Unit, Cardiff).

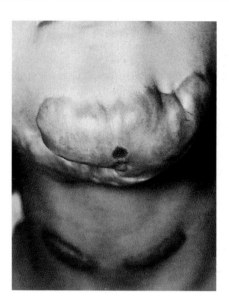

However, the most commonly encountered drugs that adversely affect healing are the corticosteroids. When taken over a long period, they suppress fibroblast and collagen synthesis.

Radiotherapy

Depending on the dosage of radiotherapy used, wounds in the immediate vicinity of the treated area may fail to heal or heal slowly. Long-term weakness of the skin and other tissue can occur following radiotherapy (Goldberg & McGinn-Byer 1997).

Abnormal scarring

Hypertrophic and keloid scarring are types of abnormal scarring caused by excessive collagen formation. In these scars the collagen fibre organization differs from that seen in normal scar. Hypertrophic scars have nodular structures, whereas keloids do not (Ehrlich & Gottrup 1998).

Hypertrophic scars **Hypertrophic** scars (Figure 1.9) are more common in the young, following traumatic injuries and large burns. In surgical wounds they tend to follow the line of the incision and occur shortly after injury. Prolonged or disrupted cytokine activity following the inflammatory phase of healing has been proposed by O'Kane (2002) as the stimulus for hypertrophic scar formation. The nodular structure of hypertrophic scars can be likened to that of an onion skin, where the collagen is arranged in parallel sheets (Ehrlich & Gottrup 1998). The collagen within the centre of the nodule is characterized by the presence of fine, disorganized fibrils, much like the collagen organization in early granulation tissue. Careful placing of incisions along Langer's lines

Figure 1.10
Keloid scarring (reproduced with kind permission from Dr C Lawrence, Wound Healing Research Unit, Cardiff).

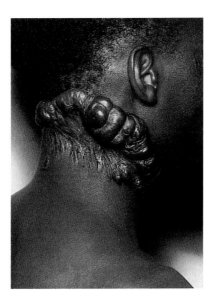

(Leaper & Gottrup 1998) and fine, absorbable suture material can often avoid excessive scar formation.

Keloid scars **Keloid** scars often occur some time after healing. They are characterized by scar tissue around the site of the wound (Figure 1.10). This is due to an increase in collagen synthesis and lysis and is also thought to be linked to the melanocyte-stimulating hormone (Eisenbeiss 1998) and it is very common in people with pigmented skin. Keloids lack the nodular structure of hypertrophic scars. Here, collagen fibres are arranged in thick bands comprising numerous fine collagen fibrils that run parallel to each other (Ehrlich & Gottrup 1998). Often these scars are larger than the wound itself and even following excision, the scar is likely to recur.

Atrophic scars Atrophic scars are weak and thin and resemble stretch marks. Although there is little to explain why they occur (as with the other abnormalities), they are more common in certain individuals than others.

Contractures

Contractures occur when there is excessive wound contraction and are most common in skin not tethered to underlying deep fascia or other structures. They often occur over joints, impairing their mobility (Iocono et al 1998). Fibroblasts constrict the neighbouring collagen fibres surrounding them (Cho & Hunt 2001), causing contracture of the tissue. Again, it is not fully understood why this occurs in some people and not others but it is important when planning surgical procedures to consider the effect of contraction, especially in areas around the joints.

LOCAL WOUND ASSESSMENT

Accurate assessment of a wound depends on the nurse's ability to recognize normal and abnormal healing. In addition, understanding the aetiology and

Table 1.3
Suture materials

Suture materials	Strength	Tissue reaction
Absorbable:		
Dexon, Maxon, Vicryl, PDS Polyglactin 910	+++	+
Gut	+	+++
Non-absorbable:		
silk, cotton	+	+++
Goretex, Ethilon, Polybutester, Tricron, Prolene	++	+
paper	+	+
steel	+++	++

+, weakest; +++, strongest.
PDS, polydioxanone sutures.
Reproduced with kind permission from Leaper & Gottrup (1998).

any underlying pathology will guide the nurse towards planning appropriate care. Local wound assessment includes sutured wounds healing by primary intention and granulating wounds healing by secondary intention.

Sutured wounds

In many surgical procedures the surgeon can bring the edges of the wound together by using sutures, staples and glues to effect primary closure (Leaper & Gottrup 1998). Suitable procedures are:

- clean surgical procedures
- procedures that result in little loss of tissue
- procedures where tissues can be brought together without causing tension.

The length of time a sutured wound will take to heal depends not only on the general health of the individual but also on the site of the incision. Where the sutured area has a good blood supply (e.g. wounds on the head and neck) healing may be completed within three days. Other sites may take up to 14 days. Sutures should be removed as soon as possible following healing to minimize scarring but must be left in for long enough to prevent the wound dehiscing.

A variety of suture materials are available (Table 1.3). More important than the choice of suture material, however, is the technique used for suturing (Bale & Leaper 2000). Surgeons are taught to follow these principles.

- Choose the right suture for the site of the incision, the tensile strength required and the resultant scarring.
- Use an adequate 'bite' when bringing the skin edges together. Larger 'bites' of tissue within the suture will generally result in a stronger wound.
- Choose the appropriate method of suturing. The choice includes:
  interrupted
  interrupted, mattress
  continuous, subcuticular
  continuous, blanket
  continuous, over-and-over.
- Maintain the correct distance evenly between individual sutures.

■ Ensure adequate and even tension while suturing – too slack and the wound will not be held together in close approximation, too tight and tissue death may occur.

Dressings

A great deal of debate has ensued about whether sutured wounds need to be dressed. It is usual for a simple dressing to be applied in theatre (e.g. an absorbent island dressing) and then removed 24–48 hours later but this practice has been challenged. Briggs (1996) and Holm et al (1997) have studied the effect of modern wound dressings on pain, ability to mobilize and return to normal activities. They report improvements in these domains when wounds are dressed with modern dressings (films and hydrocolloids) immediately postoperatively. In addition, films and hydrocolloid dressings have several practical advantages: the wound and the surrounding area may be observed easily without having to disturb dressings (films) and the patient can bathe.

Postoperative observations

The wound and the surrounding area should be observed at least once every 24 hours and whenever the patient complains of pain or discomfort.

In a normal, healthy, sutured wound, some degree of inflammation, swelling and redness is to be expected around 2–3 days postoperatively. This demonstrates that the wound is in the inflammatory phase of healing. However, observation should be maintained for the clinical signs of infection, which are:

■ generalized malaise and patient complaining of feeling unwell
■ pyrexia and tachycardia
■ wound beginning to discharge
■ the area surrounding the wound becoming red, sore, swollen and indurated
■ on removal of a suture, pus is discharged
■ partial wound breakdown following removal of sutures (Figure 1.11).

Granulating wounds

Exudate production

The amount of exudate an open wound produces can vary tremendously throughout the healing phase (Figure 1.12). In the immediate postoperative period, surgically created cavities can produce large amounts of wound exudate. It also follows that, generally, the larger the wound, the more fluid it is likely to produce. It is usual for exudate production to diminish throughout the healing phase as a wound becomes smaller. However, wounds will continue to ooze small amounts of exudate until complete re-epithelialization has occurred.

On the other hand, wound beds that are dry are not considered to be healthy and will need careful assessment and documentation in preparation for intervention (Figure 1.13).

Appearance of the wound bed

The appearance of the wound bed indicates both the stage of healing and the health of the wound.

Figure 1.11
Partial wound breakdown
following
cholecystectomy.

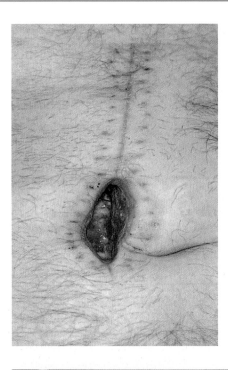

Figure 1.12
Excessive exudate being
produced by a large sacral
pressure ulcer. Note the
maceration of the skin
surrounding the wound.

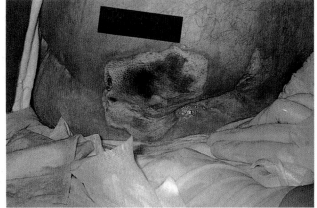

Figure 1.13
A dry wound bed on an
abdominal wall wound.

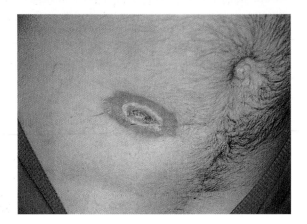

Figure 1.14
Pregranulation. An abdominal wound three days after surgery.

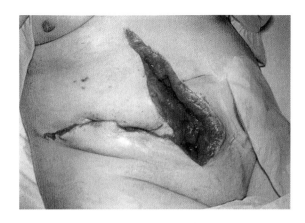

Figure 1.15
Epithelialization.

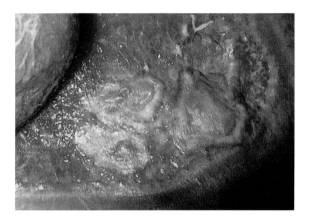

A newly created surgical cavity often appears red and raw and has adipose tissue or muscle at the base of the wound. This appearance is normal during the first two weeks of healing, prior to granulation tissue being formed (Figure 1.14).

Healthy granulation tissue appears at around 14 days and persists throughout the healing phase. It is pale pink or yellow and has a bumpy or 'cobblestone' appearance. Healthy granulation tissue is firm to touch, painless and does not bleed.

Towards the end of healing, new epithelium covers the surface of the wound. It is pale pink in colour and is usually seen at the edges of the wound, gradually creeping toward the middle to cover the wound completely (Figure 1.15).

Slough

Slough is most commonly seen lining the base of chronic wounds such as leg ulcers and pressure ulcers (Figure 1.16). It is yellow, white or grey in appearance and consists of dead, devitalized tissue, fibrin, bacteria, leucocytes, cell debris, serous exudate and deoxyribonucleic acid (Ramundo & Wells 2000).

Figure 1.16
Sloughy tissue on the wound bed of a grade IV pressure ulcer with underlying extensive tissue damage.

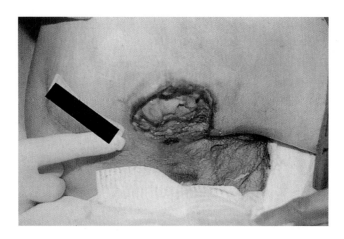

Figure 1.17
Necrotic tissue covering a pressure ulcer on the inner aspect of the knee.

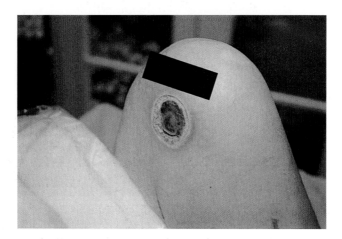

Slough may cover the wound bed totally or partially, with patches of healthy tissue. It can be dry or moist and is characterized by being firmly adherent to the base of the wound.

Necrotic tissue

Necrotic tissue is often seen in conjunction with slough. Necrotic tissue is black or blackish green in appearance and, like slough, consists of dead tissue, commonly associated with chronic wounds (Figure 1.17). Necrotic tissue can be hard and leathery in appearance or soft and moist. As with slough, it is firmly stuck to the wound bed and consists of desiccated, compressed layers of tissue. Typically, softer necrosis is associated with dead subcutaneous tissue and muscle and skin death with thicker, more leathery necrosis (Bates-Jensen 1998a). It has been argued that necrotic tissue delays or prevents healing because not only is it a physical barrier to granulation, contraction and resurfacing but it is also a medium that promotes pathogenic bacterial growth (Ayello et al 2004, Robson 1997).

Figure 1.18
An infected venous leg ulcer showing unhealthy granulation tissue and maceration of the surrounding skin.

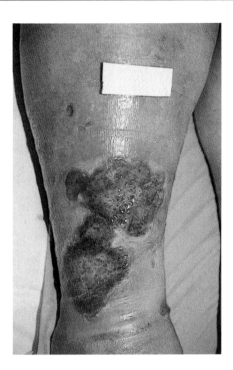

Hypergranulation

Occasionally re-epithelialization fails to take place owing to the presence of excessive granulation tissue (**hypergranulation** or proud flesh). Epithelial migration cannot continue over hypergranulation and this tissue needs to be flattened to effect complete healing through re-epithelialization.

Wound shape

It is important to recognize the importance of wound shape and its effect on healing. Ideally, surgically created cavities should be boat shaped or saucer shaped, with evenly sloping sides. This allows free drainage of wound secretions and enables easy dressing of the wound. Many chronic wounds, especially pressure ulcers, are irregularly shaped with undermining pockets, tracts and sinuses. Where these are present, drainage of wound secretions is inadequate, encouraging wound infection. Poor wound shape also restricts the range of dressing materials that can be used. Occasionally wound shape is so poor and progress towards healing is so slow that surgical revision may be needed to give the wound more regular contours.

Wound size

Generally, the larger the wound, the longer it will take to heal so it is possible, in some wound types, to predict when wounds of a given size should heal. This is possible for pilonidal sinus excisions and abdominal wall wounds (Marks et al 1983).

Wound size can be difficult to measure accurately and there are several methods of doing this. Measurement of the wound can help in the evaluation of healing (see Chapter 10).

Wound infection

Wound infection can occur at any time during the healing phase and all types of wound can become infected (Figures 1.18, 1.19). All wounds are colonized

Figure 1.19
Infection occurring during healing of a pilonidal sinus wound. Note the unhealthy appearance of the granulation tissue. An anaerobic organism has been cultured from this wound.

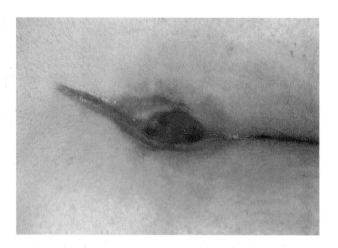

with **bacteria** that do not necessarily delay or affect healing; however, pathogenic organisms growing in large numbers are likely to produce wound infection (Leaper & Harding 2000a). Some patients are more vulnerable to infection than others and it is the relationship between the susceptibility of the host and the virulence of the pathogen that dictates the severity of the infection (Williams & Leaper 1998).

Pathogenic organisms that commonly cause wound infection are listed below.

Aerobic bacteria

Aerobic bacteria thrive in the presence of oxygen but do not necessarily depend upon it.

- *Staphylococcus aureus* is carried by around 30% of the population and causes many hospital-acquired wound infections.
- *Staphylococcus epidermidis* is found in large quantities on the intact skin of individuals. It is present in the air and in dust, being constantly shed by the skin and counts are especially high when people are frequently moving around in enclosed spaces.
- Methicillin-resistant *Staphylococcus aureus* (MRSA) has been a cause of hospital-acquired infection for many years. With the discovery of penicillin, serious outbreaks of hospital-acquired infections were brought under control. Unfortunately, *Staph. aureus* quickly developed resistance to penicillin. The emergence of MRSA was reported in 1961 (Jevans 1961) and it has been causing problems ever since (Siu 1994, Williams & Leaper 1998), especially in intensive care units and elderly care wards. Methods of spread include the unwashed hands of doctors and nurses, contact with heavily contaminated families and surfaces and airborne spread from infected patients (Bates-Jensen 1998b). A high incidence of sepsis and serious complications occurs in seriously ill patients, including those who have suffered burns or who are immunocompromised (Gilchrist & Morison 1997).
- Beta-haemolytic streptococci are found in around 5% of the population and more commonly in those suffering from acute tonsillitis. In burns and plastic

Figure 1.20
Abscess excision sites infected with *Pseudomonas*. Note the blue-green discharge characteristic of *Pseudomonas*.

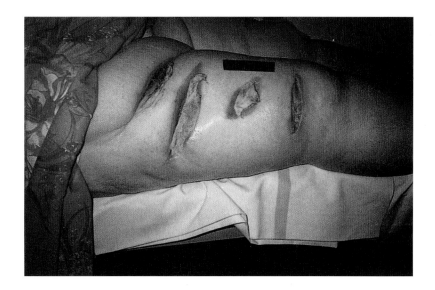

surgery units these bacteria cause infection under skin grafts and can lead to the death of the graft.

■ *Escherichia coli* and *Proteus* are normal bowel flora. These bacteria can be spread by hand contamination or by local approximation of the perineum to the wound. Sacral pressure ulcers are prime candidates for such contamination, especially if the patient is incontinent of faeces. Occasionally spillage may occur during intestinal surgery that contaminates the surgical incision.

■ *Klebsiella* and *Pseudomonas* (Figure 1.20) are found in moist conditions although they are also normal bowel commensals. Because they are free living these bacteria can easily contaminate lotions and antiseptics.

Anaerobic bacteria

Anaerobic bacteria thrive in the absence of oxygen and so are suited to the conditions found in the bowel and in soil.

■ *Bacteroides* are present in large numbers in the bowels of healthy individuals. In pilonidal sinus excisions these micro-organisms are responsible for an infection rate of around 20%, owing to the close proximity of these wounds to the anus. Leakage during bowel surgery can cause peritonitis.

■ *Clostridium welchii* is a potentially fatal organism. This spore-bearing organism is present in the bowel and in soil and when it contaminates a wound it can cause gas gangrene. Poorly perfused wound sites such as amputation stumps or deep contaminated traumatic cavities are especially at risk.

■ *Clostridium tetani* is another spore-bearing organism that infects wounds that have been exposed to dirt or soil where these bacteria are commonly found, causing tetanus in the unprotected individual.

Susceptible patients

Patients who are susceptible to developing wound infection include:

■ the immunocompromised or patients with a debilitating illness
■ patients with **devitalized** tissue in their wound (Stotts & Whitney 1999)

Figure 1.21
Sources of infection in hospital.

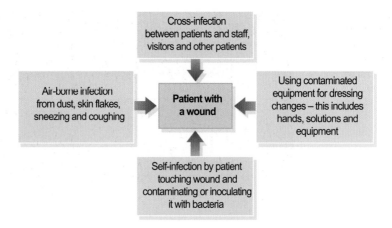

- patients with a haematoma in their wound (Leaper & Gottrup 1998)
- patients with a poor blood supply to the wound (Cooper 2000)
- patients who are at risk of contamination of their wound, e.g. through dementia or incontinence (Stotts & Whitney 1999)
- older patients – advancing age increases the risk of wound infection (Dealey 1999, Stotts & Whitney 1999)
- obese patients – gross obesity increases the risk of wound infection (Williams & Leaper 1998)
- patients who are shaved preoperatively or who stay in hospital for longer than seven days preoperatively (Cruse & Foord 1980, Dealey 1999).

Possible routes of infection in patients with wounds are shown in Figure 1.21.

Possible causes of wound infection

Wound infection does not occur in all situations where pathogenic organisms are found but depends on the number of pathogens, their virulence and the host's resistance to infection (Gardener & Frantz 2004). It occurs when the physiological balance is upset, either because the host's defences are lowered or because the micro-organism is particularly virulent (Mertz & Ovington 1993). This situation causes failure by the host to control micro-organism growth, evidenced by localized infection which, if unchecked, can lead to deep-seated and more severe infection (Gardener & Frantz 2004).

Clinical signs of infection

Infected granulation tissue (Figure 1.22) has an appearance characterized by:

- flimsy, friable granulation tissue
- superficial bridging within the wound
- spontaneous bleeding or bleeding on light contact
- pain or discomfort within the wound
- delayed healing or wound enlargement
- offensive wound exudate
- pus secretion
- **cellulitis** or inflammation in the tissues surrounding the wound (Cutting & White 2004).

Figure 1.22
A pilonidal sinus wound illustrating the clinical signs of infection (reproduced with kind permission from the *Journal of Wound Care*, London).

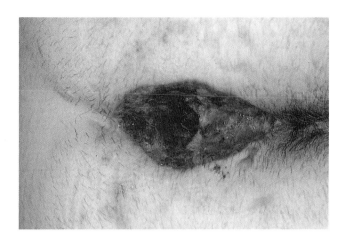

Infection in primary wound closure is characterized by:

- redness, inflammation and induration of the tissues surrounding the wound (not associated with the immediate postoperative inflammatory phase of healing, which is a normal phenomenon occurring around days 1–3 following surgery)
- partial wound breakdown accompanied by a discharge of pus or haemoserous fluid
- pain, throbbing and heat in the wound area and surrounding tissues.

It is usually necessary to take a sample of wound exudate or discharge for culture and sensitivity by the bacteriology laboratory. Identifying the organism causing the wound infection, together with its sensitivity to an antibiotic, facilitates early treatment of the wound infection.

There continues to be considerable debate regarding the best method of detecting and counting pathogenic organisms. Gilchrist and Morison (1997), Bates-Jensen (1998b) and Stotts (2000) describe a variety of methods that includes swabbing, biopsy, fine-needle aspiration and colour imaging. Most nurses are familiar with wound swabs but these are reported to be unhelpful in detecting the most pathogenic bacteria delaying wound healing (Gilchrist & Morison 1997). Nurses should consider what information they require from the laboratory and make this implicit on the laboratory forms. In addition, attention needs to be paid to swabbing technique that should include, using an aseptic technique, gathering as much exudate as possible without contaminating the sterile swab with skin flora. The swab should be sent to the laboratory as soon as possible, within 24 hours at the latest, using a transport medium where appropriate.

ASSESSMENT OF THE ENVIRONMENT

The final step in this organized approach considers the physical and social environment in which the individual is being cared for. Having a wound is likely to have a profound effect on the individual's lifestyle.

SUMMARY

This chapter has covered aspects that need to be considered when assessing any patient with a wound, whether simple or complex. Before proceeding to the next chapter, reflect on these aspects.

- **Assessment of the individual**
  Recognizing the stages of normal healing
  Recognizing abnormal healing processes
  Wound healing by primary or secondary intention
- **Factors that affect healing**
  Intrinsic
  Extrinsic
- **Assessment of the wound**
  Sutured or granulating
  Shape and size
  Infection
- **Assessment of the environment**
  Hospital based
  Community based
  Caregivers

The way in which all these aspects can be used in an organized framework is discussed in the next chapter.

FURTHER READING

Bale S, Harding K, Leaper D 2000 An introduction to wounds. Emap Healthcare Ltd, London.

Bryant R A 2000 Acute and chronic wounds: nursing management Mosby, St Louis, Missouri.

Falanga V 2001 Cutaneous wound healing. Martin Dunitz, London.

Leaper D, Harding K 1998 Wounds: biology and management. Oxford Medical Publications, Oxford.

REFERENCES

Ayello A E, Baranoski S, Kerstein M D, Cuddigan J 2004 Wound debridement. In: Wound care essentials: practice principles. Lippincott Williams and Wilkins, Springhouse, Pennsylvania.

Bale S, Leaper D 2000 Acute wounds. In: An introduction to wounds. Emap Healthcare Ltd, London.

Bale S, Morison M 1997 Patient assessment. In: Morison M, Moffatt C, Bridel-Nixon J, Bale S (eds) Nursing management of chronic wounds. Mosby, London.

Bates-Jensen B M 1997 The pressure sore status tool – a few thousand assessments later. Advanced Wound Care 10(5): 65–73.

Bates-Jensen B M 1998a Management of necrotic tissue. In: Sussman C, Bates-Jensen B M (eds) Wound care: a collaborative practice manual for physical therapists and nurses. Aspen, Gaithersburg, Maryland.

Bates-Jensen B M 1998b Management of exudate and infection. In: Sussman C, Bates-Jensen B M (eds) Wound care: a collaborative practice manual for physical therapists and nurses. Aspen, Gaithersburg, Maryland.

Briggs M 1996 Surgical wound pain: a trial of two treatments. Journal of Wound Care 5(10): 456–460.

Cho M, Hunt T K 2001 The overall approach to wounds. In: Falanga V (ed) Cutaneous wound healing. Martin Dunitz, London.

Cooper D M 2000 Assessment, measurement and evaluation: their pivotal roles in wound healing. In: Bryant R A (ed) Acute and chronic wounds: nursing management. Mosby, St Louis, Missouri.

Cruse P J E, Foord R 1980 The epidemiology of wound infection: a 10 year prospective study of 62,939 wounds. Surgical Clinics of North America 60(12): 27–40.

Cutting K F 2004 Exudate: composition and functions. In: White R J (ed) Trends in wound care, vol III. Quay Books, Salisbury.

Cutting K F, White R J 2004 Criteria for wound infection by criteria. In: White R J (ed) Trends in wound care, vol III. Quay Books, Salisbury.

Dealey C 1999 The management of patients with wounds. In: The care of wounds. Blackwell, Oxford.

Dickerson J 1995 The problem of hospital induced malnutrition. Nursing Times 92(4): 44–45.

Ehrlich H P, Gottrup F 1998 Experimental models in wound healing. In: Leaper D J, Harding K G (eds) Wounds: biology and management. Oxford Medical Publications, Oxford.

Eisenbeiss W, Peter F W, Bakhtiari C, Frenz C 1998 Hypertrophic scars and keloids. Journal of Wound Care 7(5):255–257.

European Pressure Ulcer Advisory Panel 2003 EPUAP Guidelines on the Role of Nutrition in Pressure Ulcer Prevention and Management. EPUAP Review 5(2): 50–53.

Gardener S E, Frantz R A 2004 Wound bioburden. In: Wound care essentials: practice principles. Lippincott, Williams and Wilkins, Springhouse, Pennsylvania.

Gilchrist B, Morison M 1997 Wound infection. In: A colour guide to the nursing management of chronic wounds. Mosby, London.

Goldberg M T, McGinn-Byer P 1997 Oncology-related skin damage. In: Sussman C, Bates-Jensen B M (eds) Wound care: a collaborative practice manual for physical therapists and nurses. Aspen, Gaithersburg, Maryland.

Gray D, Cooper P 2001 Nutrition and wound healing: what is the link? Journal of Wound Care 10(3): 86–89.

Hart J 2002 Inflammation 2: its role in the healing of chronic wounds. Journal of Wound Care 11: 245–249.

Holm C, Pederson J, Gronbaek F, Gottrup F 1997 Occlusive versus dry wound healing: a prospective randomised study in abdominal surgery patients. In: Leaper D, Cherry G W, Dealey C et al (eds) Proceedings of the 6th European Conference on Advances in Wound Management. Macmillan Magazines Ltd, London.

Hunter J A A 1995 Clinical dermatology, 2nd edn. Blackwell Science, Oxford.

Iocono J A, Ehrlich H P, Gotrupp F, Leaper D J 1998 The biology of healing. In: Leaper D J, Harding K G (eds) Wounds: biology and management. Oxford Medical Publications, Oxford.

Jevans M P 1961 'Celbenci'-resistant staphylococcus. British Medical Journal 1: 124.

Keicolt-Glaser J 1995 Slowing of wound healing by psychological stress. Lancet 346(8984): 1194.

Kindlen S, Morison M 1997 The physiology of wound healing. In: Morison M, Moffatt C, Bridel-Nixon J, Bale S (eds) Nursing management of chronic wounds. Mosby, London.

Leaper D J, Gottrup F 1998 Surgical wounds. In: Leaper D J, Harding K G (eds) Wounds: biology and management. Oxford Medical Publications, Oxford.

Leaper D J, Harding K G 2000a The problems of wound infection. In: An introduction to wounds. Emap Healthcare Ltd, London.

Leaper D J, Harding K G 2000b Factors affecting wound healing. In: An introduction to wounds. Emap Healthcare Ltd, London.

Lingen M W, Nickoloff B J 2001 Role of immunocytes, cytokines and angiogenesis in wound healing. In: Falanga V (ed) Cutaneous wound healing. Martin Dunitz, London.

Marks J, Hughes L E, Harding K G, Campbell H, Ribeiro C D 1983 Prediction of healing time as an aid to the management of open granulating wounds. World Journal of Surgery 7: 41–45.

Martin P 1997 Wound healing: aiming for perfect skin regeneration. Science 276: 75.

McLaren S M G 1992 Nutrition and wound healing. Journal of Wound Care 1(3): 45–55.

McLaren S 1997 Nutritional factors in wound healing. In: Morison M, Moffat C, Bridel-Nixon J, Bale S (eds) Nursing management of chronic wounds, 2nd edn. Mosby, London.

McWhirter J P, Pennington C 1994 Incidence and recognition of malnutrition in hospital. British Medical Journal 308: 945–948.

Meaume S, Merlin L, Ramamonjisoa M 1994 Major risk factors associated with pressure sores in geriatric patients. A study of 87 hospitalised elderly people with decubitus ulcers. In: Cherry G N, Leaper D J, Lawrence J C, Milward P (eds) Proceedings of 4th European Conference on Wound Management. Macmillan, London.

Mertz P M, Ovington L G 1993 Wound healing microbiology. Dermatology Clinics 11(4): 739–747.

Neal M 2001 Angiogenesis: is it the key to controlling the healing process? Journal of Wound Care 10: 281–287.

O'Kane S 2002 Wound remodelling and scarring. Journal of Wound Care 11(8): 296–297.

Padgett D, Marucha P, Sheridan J 1998 Restraint stress slows cutaneous wound healing in mice. Brain, Behavior and Immunity 12: 64.

Pinchcofsky-Devin G 1994 Nutritional wound healing. Journal of Wound Care 3(5): 231–234.

Robson M 1997 Wound infection: a failure of wound healing caused by an imbalance of bacteria. Surgical Clinics of North America 77(3): 637.

Rojas A I, Phillips T J 2001 Venous ulcers and their management. In: Falanga V (ed) Cutaneous wound healing. Martin Dunitz, London.

Ramundo J, Wells J 2000 Wound debridement. In: Bryant R A (ed) Acute and chronic wounds: nursing management. Mosby, St Louis, Missouri.

Rodgers S E 1999 The patient facing surgery. In: Alexander M F, Fawcett J N, Runciman P J (eds) Nursing practice: hospital and home, the adult. Churchill Livingstone, Edinburgh.

Siana J E, Rex S, Gottrup F 1989 The effect of cigarette smoking on wound healing. Scandinavian Journal of Plastic and Reconstructive Surgery 23: 207–209.

Siana J E, Frankild B S, Gottrup F 1992 The effect of smoking on tissue function. Journal of Wound Care 1(2): 37–41.

Siu A C K 1994 Methicillin-resistant *Staphylococcus aureus*: do we just have to live with it? British Journal of Nursing 3(15): 753–759.

Slavin J 1999 Wound healing: pathophysiology. Surgery 17(4): I–V.

Steed D 1997 The role of growth factors in wound healing. Surgical Clinics of North America 77: 575.

Stephens P, Thomas D W 2002 The cellular proliferative phase of the wound repair process. Journal of Wound Care 11: 253–261.

Stotts N 2000 Nutritional assessment and support. In: Bryant R A (ed) Acute and chronic wounds: nursing management. Mosby, St Louis, Missouri.

Stotts N, Whitney JD 1990 Nutritional intake and status of clients in the home with open surgical wounds. Journal of Community Nursing 7(2): 77–86.

Stotts N A, Whitney J D 1999 Identifying and evaluating wound infection. Home Healthcare Nurse 17(3): 159–165.

Stotts N A, Wipke-Tevis D 1997 Co-factors in impaired wound healing. In:Kransner D, Kane D (eds) Chronic wound care: a clinical source handbook for healthcare professionals. Health Management Publications,Wayne, PA.

Waldrop J, Doughty D 2000 Wound-healing physiology. In: Bryant R A (ed) Acute and chronic wounds: nursing management. Mosby, St Louis, Missouri.

Whitby D J 1995 The biology of wound healing. Surgery 13(2): 25–28.

White R J 2001 Managing exudate. Nursing Times 97(9): XI-XIII.

Witte M, Barbul A 1997 General principles of wound healing. Surgical Clinics of North America 77: 509.

Williams L 2002 Assessing patients' nutritional needs in the wound-healing process. Journal of Wound Care 11(6): 225–228.

Williams N A, Leaper D J 1998 Infection. In: Leaper D J, Harding K G (eds) Wounds: biology and management. Oxford Medical Publications, Oxford.

Wysocki A B 2000 Anatomy and physiology of skin and soft tissue. In: Bryant R A (ed) Acute and chronic wounds: nursing management. Mosby, St Louis, Missouri.

Assessing and planning individualized care

INTRODUCTION

Assessing a patient with a wound can prove to be difficult, especially for the inexperienced practitioner.

There are many ways in which nurses assess their patients: some haphazardly, some using a medical model framework and others using a nursing model. In order to use a nursing model, nurses must understand the basis of the model. In the right circumstances nursing models can provide a clear framework for practitioners to follow as well as providing an optimum level of care for the patient.

This chapter explains the theory that underpins nursing models and discusses the type of patient they might be best suited for.

When using an organized framework to identify patient problems, it is important that clear goals and outcomes are identified. The setting of goals and outcomes is explained using examples of particular wound types.

USING A NURSING MODEL TO ASSESS INDIVIDUALS

Before using a nursing model, it is important that the nurse understands the nursing theory that underpins it. Often this vital step is overlooked, as models are frequently introduced via the curriculum of a college of nursing or on a regional basis throughout all the clinical areas within an NHS trust. This only fuels the resistance to using a model, as nurses fail to understand the philosophy behind the model or its relevance to practice.

Theoretical basis of models

It is difficult in the early stages of a nursing career to understand what 'nursing' is all about. Since the introduction of nursing models, the health-care system has undergone numerous changes along with nursing practice and the role of the nurse. However, one of the major complaints still heard from practitioners is that often nursing theory has little or no relevance to clinical practice. Because models are often imposed or dictated, nurses do not have the flexibility to discover how a model fits into their line of practice or which model might be most useful.

However, nursing models can still help nurses develop a shared understanding of nursing theory that relates to their everyday clinical practice .

It could be said that the focus of nursing has always been patient need, an issue that was addressed in *The Patient's Charter* (DoH 1995). Nursing models have always focused on the patient's role in the decision-making process and emphasized the nursing rather than medical role of care.

It is within this context of an ever-changing health-care delivery system that there is a need for nursing models to develop nursing practice.

Of equal importance is the relationship between the use of models and the nursing process (Alfaro 1999). The nursing process, a system of individualized nursing care, is achieved with the use of a nursing model – it is not a nursing model itself and this distinction must be made clear (Aggleton & Chalmers 2000). So, how can the application of a nursing model help to decrease the gap between theory and practice?

Wound management is so obviously a practical subject that it can be used as a focus for the use of a model while drawing continually on the biological and behavioural scientific knowledge that underpins its practice (Figure 2.1). Using a model as a framework can help students and inexperienced practitioners bring structure into what may appear to be a bewildering array of theories, abstract concepts, haphazard treatment and intuitive behaviour. However, models are constructed on the assumption that patient-centred care is in use (Kershaw & Salvage 1986) and even where the 'named nurse' system is apparently functioning, staff shortages and heavy workload will result in a degree of task allocation. This is confusing to students who may construe this situation as the model not working, hence contributing to the 'theory–practice gap' (Cook 1991). In certain circumstances the model may need to be set aside in favour of a system that prioritizes patients' needs, which are assessed and

Figure 2.1
Wound management theory (adapted with kind permission from Akinsanya 1984).

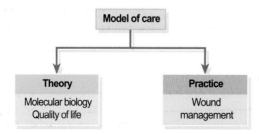

planned on a less formal basis. This informal method of care is often practised by 'experienced' nurses who feel they do not need a designated model but set their own framework through which they practise. This informal, unsystematic way of working is very difficult to pass on to others as it is often based on intuitive and ritualistic care that has little theoretical foundation (Walsh & Ford 1989).

Theories and models of nursing address four concepts:

- the individual
- society or the environment of care
- health
- nursing, its nature and role (Perry & Jolley 1991).

Deductive or inductive approach

Models are based on either a deductive or an inductive approach. These terms are derived from the physical sciences, as is the concept of using models, which originally were physical representations of physical objects. Later on, the behavioural sciences adopted the use of models to predict behaviour.

The laws of physical science were established through the formulation of hypotheses which were then formally tested by experimental methods. This is known as the deductive method; it relies heavily on controlling the variables under study and is not always suitable for the behavioural sciences such as psychology and sociology. During the 1960s sociologists found that the generation of theory was better achieved by observation of practice and behaviour. This is the inductive approach to theory generation which has been found to be very suitable to nursing studies. It also facilitated the move away from the medical model of care, as medical knowledge is largely based on the deductive method of theory generation. This shift has not been an easy or comfortable move for many nurses and often nursing models are still used as medical models. This is highlighted in Table 2.1, which is an example of the Roper activities of living model (Roper et al 1996) in use on a medical ward. The problems identified are largely medical conditions and symptoms, such as renal failure and dehydration, and it is this framework that is used by the ward nurses.

Classification of models

Models can be classified according to their underpinning theory, as follows:

- developmental
- systems
- interaction.

However, many models will not be totally illuminated by one underlying philosophy but will contain aspects of two or even all three theories. This can often lead to confusion when trying to establish the theoretical underpinnings of a particular model. The models used in this book are categorized according to their *primary* focus.

Developmental models

Developmental models focus on theories of development or change (Kershaw & Salvage 1986). These theories centre around how a person is developing and how nursing can help when normal development is threatened or impaired.

Table 2.1
A patient's problems.
Activities of living have
been grouped according
to their degree of
correspondence to
physiological systems. (P)
indicates a potential
problem (reproduced
with kind permission from
Roper et al 1983)

Activity of living	Problem statements
Maintaining a safe environment	Risk of self-injury (P)
Communicating	Diminished verbal response Anxiety, depression Accent
Breathing	Cough Infected sputum Pain Dyspnoea Cigarette smoking
Eating and drinking	Anorexia Dehydration Poor dentition Oral infection (P)
Elimination	Renal failure (P) Renal infection (P) Constipation (P)
Personal cleansing and dressing	Inability or unwillingness to care for self Excessive perspiration
Controlling body temperature	Dehydration (P)
Mobilizing	Immobility Pressure sores (P) Deep vein thrombosis Exacerbation of chest infection
Working and playing Expressing sexuality Sleeping	
Dying	Non-acceptance of nature of disease (P)

In the developmental process, stages follow a predictable course and proceed in an orderly fashion, even towards illness or death (Pearson et al 1998). Development covers not just the physical but psychological and social processes as well. Developmental models focus on helping the patient attain new developmental goals or reestablishing a developmental stage from which the patient has regressed. The two best-known models in this category are those of Peplau (1952) and Orem (1995).

Peplau's model   Hildegard Peplau was one of the first American theorists to address the changing needs of nursing (Peplau 1952). She recognized that often the care that a patient *needs* may well be different from what the patient *wants*.

Believing that nursing was based on the formation of a relationship between nurse and client, she stressed the importance of the roles and phases through which nurse and patient pass during the interpersonal process. The first purpose of the nurse is to ensure survival of the patient, the second is to help them understand and come to terms with their health problems. For example, when a patient with diabetes mellitus has a foot amputated because of ischaemia, the first concern of the nurse is control of the diabetes and infection. Both conditions, unchecked, are life threatening. The nurse's second concern is to help the patient come to terms with the loss of a foot and learn how to mobilize again.

In moving towards health, the patient experiences four phases: orientation, identification, exploration and resolution. These four phases correspond to the four phases of the nursing process.

- *Orientation* (assessment): nurse learns the nature of the difficulty the patient is experiencing; development of mutual trust; problem identification.
- *Identification* (planning): recognition by the patient of the formulation of the nurse–patient relationship; nurse plans appropriate intervention.
- *Exploitation* (implementation): patient recognizes and responds to services offered by the nurse; interpersonal relationship is fully established; both nurse and patient move towards mutual goals.
- *Resolution* (evaluation): health problem resolved or improved; nursing input no longer required or at minimal level; patient returns to independence; new goals or existing developmental stage re-established.

Peplau's model has no particular framework or form of record keeping to be used during the assessment phase. She advocates the use of the acronym SOAP:

S – the *subjective experience* as described by the patient
O – *objective observation* made by the nurse
A – *formal assessment* and identification of problems (based on S and O)
P – *plan* of action.

For an example, look at Case study 4.3.

Orem's self-care model Orem's framework has been classified previously as a systems model (Riehl & Roy 1980) and latterly as a self-care model (Aggleton & Chalmers 2000, Pearson et al 1998, Riehl-Sisca 1989). However, Fawcett (1989) and Walsh (1991) agreed that Orem's model demonstrates strong characteristics of a developmental model. The model emphasizes the concept of self-care where people take responsibility for their own health care, which is provided where possible by friends and family. The model rejects the passive role of the patient and is more in tune with today's nursing, which allows patients to participate in their own care.

The characteristics of growth, development and maturation are classified in Orem's model as self-care requisites and can be described as basic human needs. They are:

- sufficient intake of air
- sufficient intake of water
- sufficient intake of food
- satisfactory eliminatory functions
- activity balanced with rest
- time spent alone balanced with time spent with others
- prevention of danger to self
- being normal.

Two further self-care requisites are described.

- *Developmental self-care requisites:* these may affect the universal self-care requisites according to the stage of development of the individual or the environment in which the individual lives.
- *Health deviation self-care requisites:* ill health or disability may necessitate a change in self-care behaviour.

Self-care is possible when individuals are able to cope with the demands placed upon them. When these demands become too great or the individual's ability to cope decreases, then an imbalance occurs, causing a 'self-care deficit'.

Assessment using Orem's model should be carried out in two stages.

Stage 1 – establishing *if* there is a self-care deficit.

Stage 2 – if there is, establishing *why* there is a self-care deficit. Is it because the patient lacks knowledge, skill or motivation or has a limited range of behaviour?

Having identified a self-care deficit, the nurse should plan – with the patient where possible – the goals of care. The nurse must decide whether the intervention will be:

- wholly compensatory, i.e. the nurse acts for the patient completely
- partly compensatory, i.e. certain aspects of care are shared by patient and nurse
- educative-developmental, i.e. the nurse gives the patient the necessary knowledge or skills to allow self-care.

The level at which the patient is involved in planning care will depend on the patient's physical and mental state but the nurse should always aim to maximize the patient's input where possible. The patient's relatives or carers should be included in this planning as they may be a key factor in helping the patient achieve this potential.

Nursing *intervention* follows the planning stage. Orem has distinguished five methods of implementing the care plan:

1. acting or doing for another
2. guiding another
3. supporting another, physically or psychologically
4. providing an environment that promotes personal development
5. teaching another.

The move from dependence to independence is clear in this model. It must be stressed, however, that giving a patient a task to do without assessing their potential is not self-care and may have dire consequences, as in Case study 2.1. With proper assessment and planning this situation could have been avoided. Can you see why it occurred?

Systems models

Systems models are characterized by the progression along a lifespan, the examination of the system, its parts and their relationship with each other at a given time.

The major features of systems models are the system and its environment. It is how the system reacts to the environment and maintains its equilibrium

Case study 2.1

Mr Steven Jones is a 22-year-old student who has undergone surgery for excision of a pilonidal sinus. He is anxious to return home and to his studies as he has examinations in six weeks' time.

The nurse explains verbally how he can change his foam dressing himself. She does not:

- enquire if he has a carer (partner or parent) who could assist with the dressing change
- explain the importance of cleansing his foam 'bung' twice daily
- watch Steven doing the dressing change before discharge
- explain the importance of personal hygiene
- give any written explanation.

Steven goes home with his dressings but without support at home and without any kind of written guidance, he quickly forgets what he has to do. He consequently rings his general practitioner who sends the district nurse to the house to help with the dressing change. The district nurse is annoyed with Steven and the hospital as she feels this to be an unnecessary call, when she has many less able patients to call on. Steven feels stupid and inadequate that he is unable to cope.

that is of major interest. In contrast to developmental models, change is of secondary importance. Systems models are concerned with maintaining a balance along the lifespan; although each part is studied separately, interaction of the parts is most important (Pearson et al 1998).

'System' and 'environment' are defined according to the context of study, e.g. a system could be a person whose parts are body organs and whose environment is the family.

Systems may be open or closed. An open system is one of continuous inflow and outflow, the outflow becoming the inflow for the next stage of the system and so on. Open systems are therefore influenced by internal and external factors; the less interference from either of these factors, the more smoothly the system will run.

As in the human body, a disturbance in the function of one of the internal subsystems or external factors will produce an imbalance. In order for the body to maintain homeostasis, a new balance has to be achieved. This may be self-regulated, for example the production of insulin for the conversion of glucose to give energy. Outside intervention from medical and nursing staff will be required when the body is unable to regulate an imbalance; for example, when a patient has a wound infection, the initial reaction by the body will be an increase in the number of white blood cells (i.e. a lymphatic response) and also a cardiovascular response, producing the signs and symptoms of infection. With the output the patient experiences pain, which subsequently becomes an input (Figure 2.2).

Understanding this systems approach will help the nurse to identify priorities of care and provide intervention that will minimize further complications

Figure 2.2
Wound infection – a systems approach. WBC, white blood cell count; TPR, temperature, pulse, respiration (adapted with kind permission from Chapman 1985).

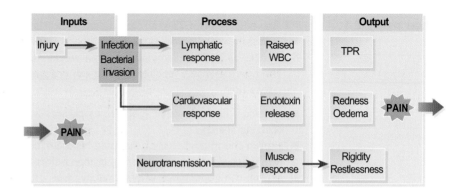

or deterioration. This method of care is proactive rather than reactive, i.e. it deals with a problem before it arises rather than after.

Two models that have a distinct systems approach are Roy's adaptation model (Roy & Andrews 1999) and Roper, Logan and Tierney's activities of living model (Roper et al 1996).

Roy's adaptation model   Calista Roy began developing this model in the mid-1960s in California. She sees the person as an individual whose behaviour is governed by a set of interrelated biological, psychological and social systems (Aggleton & Chalmers 2000). In order to maintain a balance, individuals are in a constant state of interaction, both within themselves and in their relationship with the outside world. Demands or stressors can be anything experienced in life and how an individual copes or adapts to these will vary from person to person. It is the nurse's ability to identify stressors that will influence the patient's recovery. When the nurse is able to do this, their role should be to promote the patient's ability to adapt and cope with the new demands. However, a person's response to stressors can vary. Roy (1997) argues that this is controlled by three sets of stimuli.

- *Focal*: those immediately present for the individual
- *Contextual*: those occurring alongside the focal stimuli
- *Residual*: those occurring from past learning and its effects.

As these three types of stimuli will never occur in exactly the same way at any one time, the response or adaptation will also vary. Consider the example of a patient who attends an outpatient clinic on two occasions for a wound dressing.

Visit 1

- The clinic is busy, many patients are waiting and the room is hot (contextual stimuli).
- The nurse attending him has had no lunch break, forgets his name and cannot remember what type of operation he has had (focal stimuli).
- On his last visit the wound was infected and the doctor applied a silver nitrate stick to some overgranulation; this was extremely painful (residual stimuli).

How do you think the patient coped with this visit?

Visit 2

- The clinic is quiet, cool and calm and the patient is asked to go straight in without waiting (contextual).
- A different nurse attends this week, who addresses him by his name, appears to know all about his wound and operation and explains the procedures. The wound is healthy with no complications (focal).

Now, although the patient's residual stimulus remains the same, both focal and contextual stimuli have changed. Would you expect the same behaviour on this visit?

Roy identified four principal adaptation systems that influence behaviour.

- *Physiological system*: the body's responses to food, fluids, oxygen, circulation, temperature, sensory input, exercise and rest.
- *Self-concept system*: the view that people hold of themselves, both physically and psychologically. It is concerned with how people see their own worth, both in their own eyes and in those of others.
- *Role mastery system*: focuses on the individual's need to have a place in society: the duties and responsibilities or rights and privileges they hold.
- *Interdependency system*: the balance between dependence and independence in relationships with others. Levels of friendliness, dominance and competitiveness.

Nursing intervention will be required when there is a deficit or excess within one or more of these adaptation systems.

Assessment using Roy's model, as with other nursing models, consists of two stages. In the first stage the nurse will observe behaviour using each of the four adaptation systems as a framework. If there appears to be a problem of adaptation the nurse should move on to identify whether the factors creating this problem are focal, contextual or residual.

Planning must then identify the patient-centred goals in order of priority and the type of nursing intervention required to change either the stimuli or the patient adaptation level.

Nursing will generally concentrate on the focal stimuli as these will possibly be the primary cause of the patient's behaviour. However, this model is well suited to nurses experienced in behaviour modification and counselling techniques who have the confidence and capability to change adaptive behaviour caused by residual stimuli.

Roy's model has been used as the model of choice for patients nursed in a variety of settings, particularly in relation to changes in body image, e.g. prior to amputation (Dawson 1998) and the development of sacral pressure ulcers (Harding-Okimoto 1997).

Roper's activities of living model   Nancy Roper's original model was the result of a research project undertaken between 1970 and 1974 and was a modification of previous work on Virginia Henderson's model published in 1966 (Roper et al 1980). It was the first attempt by British nurses to use a conceptual model to form a basis of care. The focus of the model is 12 activities of living (Box 2.1); it acknowledges that all individuals are involved in activities that enable them to live and grow (Pearson et al 1998). The model embraces

---

Box 2.1 Activities of living (from Roper et al 1996)

1. Maintaining a safe environment
2. Communicating
3. Breathing
4. Eating and drinking
5. Eliminating
6. Personal cleansing and dressing
7. Controlling body temperature
8. Mobilizing
9. Working and playing
10. Expressing sexuality
11. Sleeping
12. Dying

---

the concept of an individual progressing along a continuum with varying degrees of dependence and independence, according to age and health. Movement can be in either direction and it should not be assumed that everyone can reach their full potential in all 12 activities. The key to using this model is the nurse's ability to assess the person's level of independence in each of the activities of living. Patient goals should be centred around the amount of nursing help required to move along the dependence/independence continuum.

For each activity of living listed in Box 2.1, the nurse should establish:

- what the patient can normally do
- what the patient can do now
- what the patient cannot do now
- what problems may develop.

The assessment should, where possible, involve both patient and nurse in the process of identifying actual and potential problems. Not all activities may be a cause of problems; the nurse should, as always, prioritize the goals of care.

Nursing intervention will follow three models of action, as identified by Roper:

- prevention strategies
- providing comfort (physical and mental)
- enabling the patient to seek help to take responsibility for self-care.

This model is widely used in nursing in the UK and has been criticized as following the medical model on the grounds that the activities of living are equivalent to physiological responses. However, this is largely due to this model being used in an inappropriate way through misunderstanding.

Interaction models

Interaction models emphasize the social meanings people put upon all aspects of their life and the interpersonal relationships between individuals. This study of interaction between people originates from the theory of symbolic interactionism which postulates that the importance of social life lies in providing the person with language, self-concept and role-taking ability (Blumer 1969). The major focuses of such nursing models are therefore perception, communication, role and self-concept (Fawcett 1989). The key to using this type of model is to elicit the *patient's definition* of the situation; thus the model strongly identifies the active role an individual plays in any interaction.

These models are therefore unsuited to a philosophy of care that perpetuates the notion that the patient should be passive and the nurse active. Obviously in areas such as intensive care nursing, when the patient is unconscious, the nurse's active role is necessary but in many areas of wound care, interaction with patients is a central facet of management. The most widely used model from this school of thought is the Riehl (later to become Riehl-Sisca) interaction model (Riehl 1980, Riehl-Sisca 1989).

Riehl interaction model Riehl pays particular attention to psychological and sociological systems and underplays the importance of physiological systems as the primary focus of nursing problems. She believes that the essence of good assessment is when nurses attempt to 'enter the subjective world of patients'. It is only then that the nurse is able to help a patient adopt a more appropriate behaviour or role.

Nursing problems arise when there are disturbances within one or more of the three parameters – psychological, sociological or physiological.

Riehl does not give a particular assessment framework but suggests the use of the FANCAP mnemonic (Abbey 1980) – Fluids, Aeration, Nutrition, Communication, Activity, Pain. The FANCAP system was originally designed as a teaching tool and provides a bridge between nursing science and the patient.

In the first stage of assessment the nurse ascertains if the patient is adopting a role appropriate to the present situation. If there appears to be a disturbance in role, is it due to physiological, psychological or sociological parameters?

Patient-centred goals should then be identified and activities planned for patient and nurse. Nursing intervention will centre on role playing, thus extending the range of behaviour open to the patient and increasing the nurse's understanding of the patient's problem.

The interaction model offers an approach that is very different from system or developmental models. It has been used widely in psychiatric nursing, where the emphasis is on psychological and social problems. It is unlikely to find popularity in mainstream areas of wound management but can be useful when caring for patients with factitious or self-inflicted wounds (see Chapter 6).

PLANNING INDIVIDUALIZED CARE

It is important when assessing the patient to consider the outcome or goal that is to be achieved. This is often the most difficult part of the problem-solving process, especially for the inexperienced nurse. Often goals are formulated around what the nurse is trying to achieve and not what the patient may want (Aggleton & Chalmers 2000).

Setting goals and outcomes for patients with wounds

It is essential that the aims of management are established following assessment, as without them care will lack direction and evaluation will be impossible. This is not to say that once goals have been set they can never be changed, as unforeseen events may necessitate their revision. For example, following an operation to remove her appendix, Miss Susan James, a 28-year-old secretary, wished to return to work within two weeks from the date of operation. Her plan of care stated this to be one of the goals. However, seven days postoperatively she developed a wound infection which delayed healing and necessitated **antibiotic** therapy. Therefore, following evaluation of the case at seven days it was necessary to formulate a new goal, taking into account the patient's general condition and that of the wound.

Although goal setting should be patient centred, in cases such as Susan's the nurse's professional knowledge is required to advise the patient on what is the most reasonable and safest goal. Susan may still wish to return to her employment within the original goal of 14 days but she should be advised that this may cause further complications of healing and result in delaying the final outcome of care – complete wound healing.

Distinguishing goals from outcomes

Goals and outcomes are terms that are often used interchangeably and can be confusing to students. There is no set rule as to which should be used as the definitions are similar (*Concise Oxford Dictionary* 1982):

- *Goal*: object of effort or ambition
- *Outcome*: result, visible effect.

Both refer to an end-point of care, both should be measurable and both should be evaluated against the level of care received.

It may be simpler to define them by saying that an overall outcome can be achieved by the setting of step-by-step goals. To use the analogy of a football match, the *outcome* of the match is whether the teams win, lose or draw. This outcome is dictated by the number of *goals* scored during the match. The outcome of care can be considered to be the ultimate aim of management. Whether or not it is achieved will depend on reaching step-by-step goals of care that the nurse and patient have set out for themselves.

Setting outcomes

Difficulty may be experienced when setting an outcome of management for patients with wounds because of the complexity of the wound-healing process and the different types of wounds encountered.

Acute wounds

For patients with acute wounds the outcome will normally be that of complete healing. Acute surgical wounds should heal within a predicted period without complication. Work by Marks et al (1983) demonstrated that an open granulating wound (such as excision of pilonidal sinus) will generally heal within 12–16 weeks. Therefore, when setting outcomes for a patient following this type of surgery, it is possible to be objective not only about the healing potential but also about the time in which healing should be achieved. This is a good marker for evaluation, as there should be a predictable decrease in wound size as the days to healing progress. Failure to correspond with this may indicate that all is not well with the wound-healing process.

Although acute wounds may be easier to evaluate in terms of healing time, it should be remembered that healing is not always the desired outcome; the patient may have other motives and the nurse should be aware that if a wound is not healing as predicted and there are no obvious clinical signs to account for this delay, other factors should be considered. Although difficult to prove, there is some evidence to support the theory of self-inflicted injury by some patients who have an ulterior motive for prolonging the wound (Baragwanath & Harding 1994). It is important to remember that complete healing should not be achieved at all costs, as the management and intervention used to achieve this may compromise the patient's quality of life.

Quality of life usually becomes more of an issue when dealing with patients whose wounds are long-standing and chronic.

Chronic wounds

The outcome of care for patients with a chronic wound is more difficult to plan, as often healing will not be achieved for many months or years, if at all.

Chronic wounds are formed when predisposing conditions such as diabetes impair the tissue's ability to heal the damage (Jones et al 2004). However, other factors such as proteases and proinflammatory cells have been shown to prolong the healing process (Phillips et al 1998). It is not unusual for individuals to have lived with a leg ulcer for 30 years or experienced an unhealed wound sinus for many months.

Malignant wounds will not be expected to heal and in most cases become worse; therefore the outcome of care is palliation. The prime objective is alleviation of distressing symptoms, thereby maximizing the patient's quality of life. The principle, however, remains the same; that whatever the stated outcome, it should be set against measurable and observable goals.

Setting goals   Patient goals should be defined by precise criteria, which are:

- *how well?*: the standard or degree of accuracy at which we expect the patient to perform
- *condition*: the circumstances under which the patient is to do it
- *patient response*: what is it we want the patient to be able to do? (Sparrow & Pearson 1985).

It is not always easy to write clear criteria which are also measurable and observable. It is best to avoid using subjective terms such as 'know', 'understand' and 'learn', as these do not tell us very much about how or what the patient is able to do.

Example

Edwina Banks has a venous ulcer on her right leg. She is currently having compression bandaging but the nurses would like her to complement this therapy with leg elevation.

The *outcome* of the care is to achieve complete healing of the ulcer within 4–5 months. It is necessary to formulate some patient-centred goals to achieve this. Look at the following goal: does it satisfy the three criteria outlined above?

Goal: Edwina to elevate both legs at regular intervals during the day.

This goal does not really comply with the criteria as it gives no indication of 'how well' we want Edwina to elevate her legs. The 'condition' under which she is to elevate them is not stated as she will not know how regular is regular! The only thing she knows is that it is to be achieved during the day. Only the 'patient response' is stated, which is that she is required to elevate her legs. No date is given as to when she is to achieve the goal by, therefore how will the nurses know when to evaluate if it is being achieved or not?

PRACTICE POINTS

How should this goal be written? Try to write it yourself before looking at the answer.

A more useful statement of the goal is as follows.

Goal: Edwina to elevate both legs at height above heart level for one hour in the morning and one hour in the evening by 10 March.

The goal now defines the patient response (elevation), the conditions (one hour twice a day) and 'how well?' (at a height above heart level).

Although this goal states all the criteria, unless the nurse has fully explained *why* the patient must elevate her legs and the best way this can be achieved, this goal may seem rather daunting or the patient may not realize the importance elevation plays in the healing process.

As previously stated, goals *must* be patient centred and individualized. Edwina needs to know that she can achieve this goal by lying on a sofa with her feet on the arm of the sofa; however, she may not own a sofa or may have a chest condition which prevents her from lying down. All these facts should have been ascertained during the assessment process so that this goal can be achieved by some other means.

It is still necessary to evaluate at the stated time whether Edwina has been able to achieve her goal. If not, then changes to her care programme may be required.

Planning and writing outcomes and goals can be time-consuming and difficult. They are also dependent on the practitioner's experience in deciding what is achievable for an individual patient.

SUMMARY

This chapter has outlined ways of using a nursing model when assessing patients with different wound aetiologies nursed in a variety of settings. Nursing models are used throughout the following chapters, demonstrating their practical application in the clinical setting. Make sure you have an understanding of their theoretical basis before moving on to the next chapter.

Models are classified as:

- **Developmental**
  Peplau's model (Peplau 1952)
  Orem's model (Orem 1995)
- **Systems**
  Roy's adaptation model (Roy & Andrews 1999)
  Roper, Logan and Tierney's activities of living model (Roper et al 1996)
- **Interaction**
  Riehl's interaction model (Riehl-Sisca 1989).

Remember also when assessing patients to identify measurable goals and outcomes that will provide a basis for evaluation of the patient's care.

FURTHER READING

Benner P, Wrubel J 1989 The primacy of caring. Stress and coping in health and illness. Addison-Wesley, Menlo Park, California.

Bryant R A (ed) 2000 Acute and chronic wounds. Nursing management, 2nd edn. Mosby Yearbook, St Louis, Missouri.

George J B (ed) 2002 Nursing theories: the base for professional nursing practice. Prentic-Hall, New Jersey.

Jamieson E, McCall J 1997 Clinical nursing practice. Churchill Livingstone, London.

McQuiston C M, Webb A A (eds) 1995 Foundations of nursing theory. Sage, Thousand Oaks, California.

REFERENCES

Abbey J 1980 Fancap: what is it? In: Riehl J P, Roy C (eds) Conceptual models for nursing practice, 2nd edn. Appleton-Century-Crofts, New York.

Aggleton P, Chalmers H 2000 Nursing models and nursing practice, 2nd edn. Macmillan, London.

Akinsanya J A 1984 The use of theories in nursing. Nursing Times 80(14): 59–60.

Alfaro R 1999 Application of the nursing process. Lippincott, London.

Baragwanath P, Harding K G 1994 The management of a patient with a factitious wound. Journal of Wound Care 3(6): 286–287.

Blumer H 1969 Symbolic interactionism: perspective and method. Prentice Hall, Englewood Cliffs, New Jersey.

Chapman C 1985 Theory of nursing: practical application. Harper and Row, London.

Concise Oxford Dictionary 1982 Oxford University Press, Oxford.

Cook S 1991 Mind the theory–practice gap in nursing education. Journal of Advanced Nursing 16: 1462–1469.

Dawson S 1998 Adult/elderly care nursing: pre-amputation assessment using Roy's adaptation model. British Journal of Nursing 7 (9): 536–542.

Department of Health (DoH) 1995 The Patient's Charter. Department of Health, London.

Fawcett J 1989 Analysis and evaluation of conceptual models of nursing, 2nd edn. F A Davies, Philadelphia.

Harding-Okimoto M B 1997 Pressure ulcers, self-concept and body image in spinal cord injury patients. SCI Nursing 14 (4): 111–117.

Jones V J, Bale S, Harding K G 2004 Acute and chronic wound healing. In: Baranoski S, Ayello E A (eds) Wound care essentials: practice principles. Lippincott, Williams and Wilkins, Springhouse, Pennsylvania.

Kershaw B, Salvage J (eds) 1986 Models for nursing. John Wiley, Chichester.

Marks J, Hughes L E, Harding K G, Campbell H, Ribeiro C D 1983 Prediction of healing time as an aid to the management of open granulating wounds. World Journal of Surgery 7: 641–645.

Orem D 1995 Nursing – concepts of practice, 5th edn. Mosby Yearbook, St Louis, Missouri.

Pearson A, Vaughan B, Fitzgerald M 1998 Nursing models for practice, 2nd edn. Heinemann, London.

Peplau H 1952 Interpersonal relations in nursing. G P Putnam, New York.

Perry A, Jolley M 1991 Nursing: a knowledge for practice. Edward Arnold, London.

Phillips T, Al-Almoudi E, Liverkus M 1998 Effect of chronic wound fluid on fibroblasts. Journal of Wound Care 7 (10): 527–532.

Riehl J P 1980 The Riehl interaction model. In: Riehl J P, Roy C (eds) conceptual models for nursing practice, 2nd edn. Appleton-Century-Crofts, New York.

Riehl J P, Roy C (eds) 1980 Conceptual models for nursing practice, 2nd edn. Appleton-Century-Crofts, New York.

Riehl-Sisca J P 1989 The Riehl interaction model. In: Riehl-Sisca J P (ed) Conceptual models for nursing practice, 3rd edn. Appleton and Lange, Norwalk, Connecticut.

Roper N, Logan W W, Tierney A J 1980 The elements of nursing. Churchill Livingstone, Edinburgh.

Roper N, Logan W W, Tierney A J 1983 Using a model for nursing. Churchill Livingstone, Edinburgh.

Roper N, Logan W W, Tierney A J 1996 The elements of nursing, 4th edn. Churchill Livingstone, Edinburgh.

Roy C 1997 Future of the Roy model: challenge to re-define adaptation. Nursing Science Quarterly 10(1): 42–48.

Roy C, Andrews H 1999 The Roy adaptation model, 2nd edn. Appleton and Lange, Stamford, Connecticut.

Sparrow S, Pearson A 1985 Teach yourself goal setting. Nursing Times 16: 34–35.

Walsh M 1991 Models in clinical nursing: the way forward. Baillière Tindall, London.

Walsh M, Ford P 1989 Nursing: rituals, research and rational actions. Butterworth-Heinemann, Oxford.

SECTION

2

Intervention

CHAPTER

3

Principles of wound interventions

KEY ISSUES   This chapter covers a whole range of interventions that will enable the reader to provide comprehensive management for patients in any range of clinical situations. The following principles are outlined.

Development of Dressing Materials
■ Historical perspective on wound management
■ Basis of moist wound healing
■ Range of modern wound dressings

Management of Sutured and Granulating Wounds
■ Signs of infection
■ Debridement
■ Exudate production

Methods to Reduce Spread of Infection
■ Use of aseptic techniques
■ Hand-washing technique

Cleansing of Wounds
■ Indications for cleansing
■ Methods of cleansing

INTRODUCTION   Wound interventions comprise a plethora of therapies that include wound dressings and topical agents, physical devices, biological substances and skin substitutes. Although such technologies make a major contribution to the management of wounds, the principles of cleansing, cross-infection and management of necrotic or infected tissue are also essential elements of wound management.

   This chapter traces the history of wound treatments that have underpinned the development of today's wound therapies. It then focuses on the basic principles and techniques of wound interventions that should inform the clinical practice of all nurses involved in wound care.

HISTORICAL PERSPECTIVE

Comprehensive historical texts on wound healing are few and far between, although wound dressings do feature in some medical textbooks (Hunter 1835, Rhodes 1986). One work worthy of mention is *The healing hand: man and wound in the ancient world* (Majno 1975, cited in Leaper 2000).

Early history

For early humans most wounds and injuries were the result of accidents and fighting. These injuries represented a life-threatening problem, with blood loss being a major factor; haemostasis was achieved using whatever materials came readily to hand, including sand, leaves and faeces.

Records that have survived include cave paintings from 25 000 years ago found in Spain, which illustrated the common wounds found in early humans, clay tablets from the Sumerians and papyrus from the Egyptians (Leaper 2000). In a history of Scandinavian folklore, Bergmark (1967) suggested that plant extracts have been used for thousands of years to treat wounds. Surgery was performed in China, Egypt and Mesopotamia and wound treatments included herbal medicines, sutures made from gum-coated linen, thorns and threads, resin, honey, lard, myrrh, milk and water (Leaper 1986).

Recognizing and treating infection

Hippocrates (460–377 BC) encouraged **suppuration** to debride devitalized tissue and to reduce inflammation (Forrest 1982). Nature, in Hippocrates' opinion, would heal wounds.

Nearer to the time of Christ, Celsus (25 BC–AD 50) wrote eight books on medicine and surgery. In *De medicina* Celsus, for the first time, clearly described the four cardinal signs of infection, though these were not specifically describing wounds: '*Nota vera inflammationis sunt quattuor; rubor et tumor cum calor et dolor*' – the signs and symptoms of redness, swelling, heat and pain. Celsus also recommended the early closure of fresh wounds and the surgical debridement of contaminated wounds.

Galen (AD 131–200) was a physician and anatomist who is thought to have produced over 500 books. His descriptions of routine wound management were typical of treatments of that time. Galen is famous for his theory of 'laudable **pus**', '*pus bonum et laudabile*', advocating that should a wound become infected and suppurate, this process should be allowed to continue. He used dung, writing ink and wine as wound treatments and also made haemostatic concoctions out of frankincense and aloes mixed with eggs and fur clippings (Dealey 2002). One of Galen's major contributions was to observe that spreading infection in a wound often resulted in widespread systemic sepsis and death (Leaper 2000). However, Galen believed that when infection localized and then discharged itself, the wound would go on to heal without problems. During the Middle Ages medical practitioners misinterpreted this message to mean that pus formation was both desirable and necessary for healthy healing. Clean, uninfected wounds were inoculated with a variety of noxious substances in order to stimulate pus formation. These practices continued from the 7th to the 14th centuries. It was not until the 19th century that Pasteur and Lister managed to persuade their colleagues that mortality rates could be reduced by using antiseptics and **aseptic** principles.

Theodoric of Lucca (1205–1298) was most famous for his skills in inducing anaesthesia using mandrake and opium-soaked sponges that were inhaled or swallowed. His contribution to wound care included his gentle approach to cleansing with honey and wine and dressing with lint soaked in warm wine (Dealey 2003).

The anonymous Wellcome Manuscript 564 (1392) gives a comprehensive account of wound care in London at this time. Naylor (1999) reviewed its contents and reports definitions of acute wounds and chronic ulcers, malignant and infected wounds. Treatments including compression bandaging, moist wound dressings, occlusive dressings, a nutritious diet and wound cleansing are described in detail in this document. Naylor (1999) also found a list of factors that prolong healing, with bullet points that cited systemic disease, impaired blood supply and unsuitable wound treatment as examples.

Andreas Vesalius (1514–1564) achieved much before the age of 29, mainly his contribution to anatomy and physiology. As with Theodoric of Lucca, he rejected the harsher treatments, using instead eggs and oil to dress wounds.

Sir Charles Bell (1774–1842) was recognized for his work during the battle of Waterloo (1815). This was an era when advances were being made in surgical technique and the development of surgical instruments. On hearing of the devastation at the battle, Bell travelled to Belgium with his assistant, to find 50 000 dead or injured men. Both sides had suffered terrible injuries and Bell operated on these men 'until his clothes were stiff with blood' and his arms so tired they were 'powerless with exertion of using the knife'. Bell and other surgeons corresponded with each other and, through these letters, it is possible to gain some understanding of the standard of surgery at this time. Surgical **debridement** was a widespread procedure, with devitalized bone and muscle excised. The control of haemorrhage was also undertaken by using ligatures and the range of surgical instruments was quite sophisticated. Many men died of their injuries through sepsis and also tetanus that, today, would be treatable.

Pasteur (1822–1895) discovered micro-organisms and bacteria, although initially his interest was not in patients with infection but in the role of bacteria in the fermentation of wines. Pasteur used his knowledge in this field to develop heat sterilization (pasteurization).

Joseph Lister (1827–1912) was born to a Quaker family in 1827 and was fortunate to have the high standard of education to which wealthy Quaker families had access. While obtaining a degree in Arts from University College, London, he developed an interest in medicine. His adulthood was hampered by physical and mental ill health and it was not until 1860 that he became a professor of surgery in Glasgow. It was here that Lister worked on aseptic principles, antiseptic treatment of wounds and the use of carbolic spray during surgical procedures. His interest was drawn to the problems related to sepsis and a high mortality rate amongst the patients in the Glasgow hospitals.

It was Lister who translated Pasteur's work to the field of patient care. Lister used Pasteur's findings to link suppuration of wounds with **septicaemia**, tetanus, gangrene and subsequent death. Although initially Lister used heat sterilization, he soon turned to chemical antiseptics. When Lister discovered how effective carbolic acid was, he was able to revolutionize surgical techniques. Infection and mortality rates fell dramatically as Lister used a combination of clean linen, a clean room, the use of carbolic acid spray and hand washing to reduce infection. Lister was a surgeon in King's College, London, for many years and for the 2702 patients under his care, the postoperative mortality rate was 2%.

The adoption of aseptic techniques

The medical staff of the 19th century remained, for many years, unconvinced of the benefits of the principles advocated by Pasteur and Lister. It was only in 1876 when Lister published *On the antiseptic principle in the practice of surgery* that his profession took notice of him. Gradually his work began to be expanded and developed, with steam sterilization used for surgical instruments and dressings. Theatre and dressing packs became available.

World War I

The introduction of aseptic technique during surgery and the use of operating theatres (as opposed to the kitchen table) brought a more controlled environment to surgery. Scrubbing-up procedures, gloves and sterile dressings were other methods being developed to reduce wound infection. Tulle gras dressings were developed as a low-adherent dressing. Carbolic acid was found to have too many side-effects so Eusol and Dakin's solution became popular. Eusol (an acronym for Edinburgh University Solution of Lime) contained chlorinated lime and boric acid diluted with water. Dakin's solution contained chlorinated lime, boric acid and sodium carbonate. Infection was a real problem in World War I, with contamination of wounds by earth and dirt being widespread, leading to gas gangrene and many subsequent deaths.

Antibiotics

The first sulphonamide, prontosil rubrum, was developed in 1936 by Domagh (1895–1964) and its use transformed the prognosis of many bacterial diseases (Rhodes 1986). However, it had severe side-effects on the kidneys and blood. By comparison, a virtually harmless antibiotic was soon to be discovered. Through his accidental discovery of penicillin, Fleming (1881–1955) revolutionized the care of many patients with infections. He found that bactericidal substances were released from *Penicillium* mould. This finding was used in the treatment of humans with infection by Howard Florey and Ernst Chain in 1941.

At the same time that Fleming was working on penicillin, Colebrook was studying the role of haemolytic streptococcus in relation to childbirth and the problems of puerperal sepsis. Colebrook discovered that sulphonamide contained in the dye prontosil was active against streptococcal infection. Subsequently Colebrook looked at the problem of streptococcal infection in burn patients. Using asepsis and antiseptics, topical penicillin cream and stringent cross-infection measures, he much improved the prognosis for burns victims. Due to his political activities, the 1952 Fireguard Act was introduced as a way of preventing burns.

Dressings and wound cleansing

Around 2500BC clay tablets in Mesopotamia recorded the use of milk and water to cleanse wounds and the application of honey or resin dressings or myrh and frankincense (Forrest 1982). Hippocrates (460–377 BC) advocated early haemostasis and the treatment of contused wounds with salves. Many years later, a French surgeon, de Mondeville (1260–1320), also used water to cleanse wounds. He recommended compress dressings of hot wine, encouraging patients to rest and eat nutritious food (Dealey 2004). However, there were many differences in treatments. In de Mondeville's time, another surgeon, de Chauliac (1300–1368), was using oily salves and mesh packing to promote pus formation.

Paracelsus (1493–1541) developed a theory that man had a juice that continually circulated round the body to keep the tissues and organs healthy and in a good state of repair. Consequently he recommended that all medicines, treatments and dressings should aim to maintain these body juices in the optimum condition. To this end he advocated the use of minerals such as salts of mercury and antimony on wounds.

Ambroise Paré (1510–1593) was the founder of military surgery in the 16th century. An advocate of the 'laudable pus' theory, his decision to stop using noxious substances to induce infection came about when the boiling oil he was using on the battlefield ran out and he used, as an alternative, egg yolks on the battle wounds of soldiers. Compared with soldiers treated with boiling oil, soldiers treated with egg yolk had a higher survival rate and Paré changed his philosophy. Subsequently, Paré said, 'I dressed his wounds, God healed him', the quote for which he is famous: '*Je le pansay, et Dieu le guarit*'. He used powder of rock alum, verdigris, Roman vitriol, rose honey and vinegar boiled together to form a wound dressing (Dealey 2004). Like de Mondeville, Paré also recommended that patients rested and ate nourishing foods.

Although German, Heister (1683–1758) was most influential in France. He described wound treatments, especially the bandages and dressings that were used. He carefully catalogued wounds in great detail, describing their size and shape, and the cocktails of dressings which were used.

Joseph Gamgee (1828–1886) qualified first as a veterinary surgeon and later studied medicine. He gained experience in the Crimean War and at the Royal Free Hospital in London, going on to work in Birmingham. It was here that Gamgee became interested in wound healing. He wrote of the need for 'utmost gentleness in dealing with wounds and infrequent changes of dressing'. Through working with cotton wool and gauze, he designed an 'absorbent and antiseptic surgical dressing'. This consisted of pads of degreased cotton wool covered in gauze that was bleached to give it absorbency. In these early days this dressing formed a barrier to cross-infection and provided a warm environment at the wound bed. Gamgee also soaked his dressing in phenol and iodine occasionally.

THE DEVELOPMENT OF MOIST WOUND HEALING

The zoologist George Winter (1927–1981) investigated wound healing in cutaneous wounds in the domestic pig. He later became interested in wound dressings and worked on covering wounds in an experimental model (using the pig) and observing healing rates. In his most famous piece of work, Winter observed that wounds covered with an occlusive dressing healed faster than those left to dry out (Winter 1962). It was from this work that the principles of moist wound healing were developed. Research in human wounds (Dyson et al 1988, Hinman & Maibach 1963) confirmed a similar acceleration in healing under moist conditions.

Under dry conditions the bed of an open wound rapidly dries out and forms a scab made up of dead and dying cells. New epidermal cells migrate in the moist environment found under the scab, so extending the healing phase. In a moist environment **exudate** bathes the wound bed with nutrients and many modern dressing materials are designed to maintain moisture. In 1985 Turner evaluated the needs of healing wounds and listed the criteria that should be fulfilled by a good wound dressing (Turner 1985). These criteria were later updated by Bale and Morison (1997).

- Non-adherent
- Impermeable to bacteria
- Capable of maintaining a high humidity at the wound site while removing excess exudate
- Thermally insulating
- Non-toxic and non-allergenic
- Comfortable and conformable
- Capable of protecting the wound from further trauma
- Requires infrequent dressing changes
- Cost-effective
- Long shelf life
- Available both in hospital and in the community

The range of modern wound dressings is outlined in Table 3.1, which lists their properties, presentation, dressing change frequency and indications. Examples of many of these dressings in use are shown in Figures 3.1–3.7.

MANAGEMENT OF SUTURED WOUNDS

The vast majority of sutured wounds heal without complication. Dressings applied in theatre need not be changed or disturbed unless there is a good reason for doing so. Dressings should be changed and the incision site observed if:

- the dressings become stained by discharge
- the clinical signs of infection are present, i.e. pain, inflammation, redness, impaired movement
- the patient shows general signs of infection.

MANAGEMENT OF OPEN OR GRANULATING WOUNDS – MANAGING THE NORMAL AND ABNORMAL

Debridement of devitalized tissue

The presence of sloughy, necrotic, devitalized tissue on the wound bed can delay healing and also increases the risk of wound infection (Figure 3.8). It is important to remove devitalized tissue as quickly and efficiently as possible to reduce the bioburden of the wound and to control or prevent infection (Ayello et al 2004). This can be difficult to achieve, however, as when both slough and necrotic tissue are firmly stuck to the wound bed and cannot simply be wiped away. There are several ways of achieving wound debridement.

Sharp debridement

Sharp debridement is by far the quickest and most effective method as debridement is immediate and a healthy wound bed can result (Figure 3.9). Here the devitalized or dead tissue is cut away from the healthy tissue using a scalpel, scissors or laser. However, the clinician undertaking this procedure must be able to differentiate between healthy and unhealthy tissue and also be knowledgeable about the anatomy of the area being debrided (Ayello et al 2004). Thorough and effective surgical debridement down to healthy, viable tissue is best undertaken by a doctor with surgical skills or a specially trained nurse, as some bleeding usually results (Ramundo & Wells 2000). In the UK

Table 3.1
The range of modern wound dressings

Dressing	Properties	Availability	Dressing change frequency	Indications
Semipermeable films e.g. Opsite, Tegaderm	Polyurethane or co-polymer with a semipermeable adhesive layer Conformable Clear dressing allows wound inspection	Sheets ranging from 5 × 5 cm to large theatre drapes	Designed to stay in place for several days. Should be changed when leakage is imminent	Primary or secondary dressing Superficial and epithelializing wounds: minor burns, Grade II pressure ulcers Postoperative dressing for sutured wounds IV line sites
Low-adherent e.g. Mepitel, Mepilex, N-A Ultra, Profore Wound Contact Layer, Tegapore	Low adherence to wound bed Allow passage of exudate through dressing	Sheets of various sizes from 5 × 5 cm	Designed to stay in place for several days. Supplementary absorbent padding can be changed more frequently without disturbing wound bed	Primary dressing Contact layer that can be used with absorbent padding
Medicated e.g. Acticoat, Aquacel AG, Contreet, Inadine, Iodoflex	Donates antimicrobial agent from dressing to wound bed Controls bacterial burden Effective against a broad spectrum of microorganisms	Variety of wound dressings Sheets and cavity dressings	When saturated, leaking or when active agent has been absorbed	Where microorganisms are adversely affecting healing Clinical signs of infection Primary dressings All wound types
Alginates e.g. Algisite, Comfeel, Seasorb, Cutinova, Kaltostat, Sorbsan, Tegagel	Highly absorbent Low adherent as gels on contact with exudate Some have haemostatic properties	Sheets of various sizes, packing and ropes	Designed to stay in place for several days Change when saturated or leaking imminent	Moderately to heavily exuding wounds of all aetiology Flat and cavity wounds, sinus tracts
Collagens e.g. Fibracol, Promogran	Mixture of collagen and oxidized regenerated cellulose. Collagen is prepared from bovine dermis as a 4% suspension Donates collagen to wound bed to stimulates cellular migration and new tissue development Non-adherent and absorbent	Sheets of various sizes	Designed to be used on debrided wounds or those where no debris is present Wounds should be free of the clinical signs of infection Usually requires a secondary dressing	Full thickness pressure ulcers, venous leg ulcers and mixed aetiology leg ulcers

Table 3.1

Continued

Dressing	Properties	Availability	Dressing change frequency	Indications
Foams e.g. 3M Foam, Allevyn, Allevyn Cavity, Biatain, Cutinova, Lyofoam, Tielle	Absorbent, conformable Atraumatic at dressing change Easy to apply and remove	Sheets of various sizes Cavity dressings Some are adhesive Some are shaped	Designed to stay in place for several days Change when saturated or leaking imminent	Moderately to heavily exuding wounds of all aetiology
Hydrocolloids e.g. Combiderm, Comfeel Plus, Granuflex (Duoderm), Tegasorb	Absorbent Hydrophilic colloid particles bound to polyurethane foam Impermeable to bacteria Some are semi-clear	Sheets of various sizes and shapes Usually adhesive Various thicknesses	Designed to stay in place for several days Change when saturated or leaking imminent	Low to moderately exuding wounds of all aetiologies Flat and cavity wounds
Hydrogels e.g. Aquaflow, Intrasite, Nu-Gel, Purilon Gel, Tegagel	Rehydrates wound bed by donating water Used to facilitate autolysis where necrotic or devitalized tissue is present Non-adherent Water or glycerine based, crossed-linked polymer that contains 80–99% water	Sachets or tubes of gel, sheets or strips	Usually require a secondary dressing to hold gel in place and to prevent evaporation of water Can be left for several days but can macerate surrounding skin if not changed frequently enough Change when leaking imminent	Dry wound beds of all aetoiologies Caution where gangrene might be mistaken for necrotic tissue (check vascular status) Not recommended for heavily exuding wounds

Figure 3.1
A semipermeable film dressing being used to treat a grade II pressure ulcer.

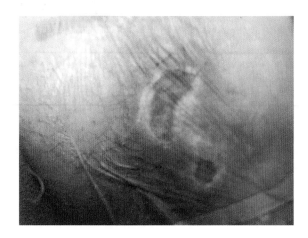

Figure 3.2
An adhesive foam dressing being used in the anal area to prevent wound contamination.

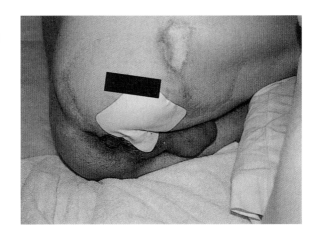

Figure 3.3
An alginate dressing used as a primary wound contact on a venous leg ulcer prior to compression therapy.

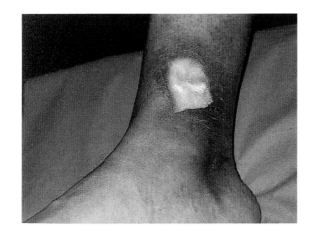

Figure 3.4
An alginate rope being packed into a cavity wound.

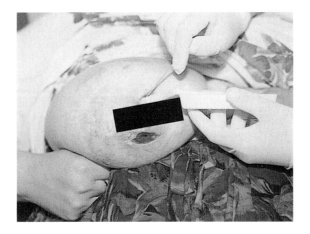

Figure 3.5
Hydrocellular foam dressing used on a heavily exuding sacral pressure ulcer (top). The dressing is held in place with a semipermeable film (below).

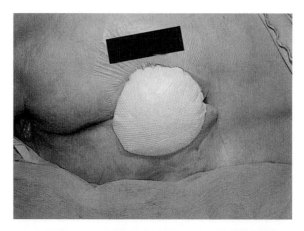

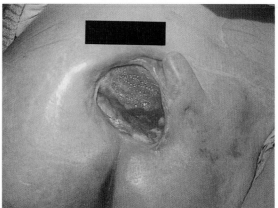

Figure 3.6
A hydrocolloid dressing following four days' treatment on an axillary wound.

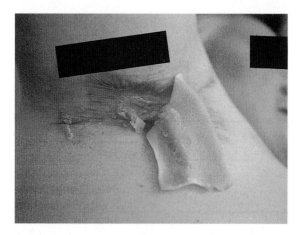

Fairbairn et al (2002) developed a framework for knowledge and competency-based practice to provide guidelines for nurses wishing to undertake sharp debridement. For some patients access to a clinician competent to perform debridement is not possible, especially when patients are being cared for in the community and a conservative approach is required.

Figure 3.7
A hydrocolloid dressing used as a primary wound contact for a venous leg ulcer.

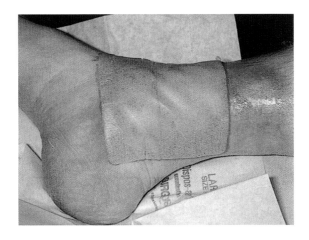

Figure 3.8
Necrotic tissue on the bed of a pressure ulcer. It may have deep tissue damage underneath.

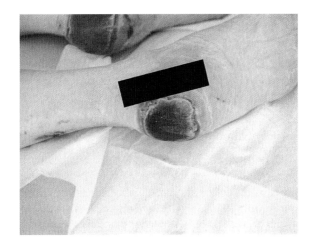

Figure 3.9
Sharp debridement of necrotic tissue.

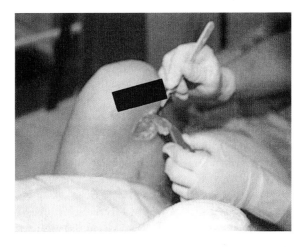

The use of modern dressing materials

Hydrogels and **hydrocolloids** effectively rehydrate devitalized tissue. In the presence of sufficient moisture, **autolysis** of devitalized tissue takes place. With prolonged use of moist dressings, the autolytic processes will facilitate separation of viable from non-viable tissue. This process occurs by the action of phagocytic cells and proteolytic enzymes that soften and liquefy necrotic tissue so that it can be digested by macrophages (Ayello et al 2004). For autolysis to proceed, a moist, vascular wound environment is required (Ramundo & Wells 2000).

Enzymatic agents

Enzymatic agents can be applied topically to wound beds containing devitalized tissue. Such enzymatic agents are sourced from fish, fruit, animals and bacteria (Ramundo & Wells 2000). They can be categorized by the tissue type they target, namely proteolytic, fibronolytic or collagenase (Ayello et al 2004). It is recommended that the skin surrounding the wound is protected by using a barrier ointment or dressing because some enzymes can damage healthy skin.

Healthy granulating and epithelializing wounds

The aim of intervention for wounds that are in the proliferative phase of healing and producing granulation tissue is to maintain an environment conducive to healing. Following assessment of the patient, the wound characteristics and the social environment of the patient, a nursing model can be selected and a wound care plan formulated.

Controlling wound exudate

Although exudate is produced by all healthy open wounds, excessive exudate may be produced by particularly large wounds or deep cavities. If exudate is not controlled, leakage may occur which soils and stains clothes and bed clothes, so causing discomfort and embarrassment. Excessive exudate can also cause maceration of the wound bed and skin surrounding the wound. It can damage skin through enzymatic activity and by causing physical damage to the structure of skin. Cutting and White (2002) argue that when patients have existing pressure ulcers, the exudate that drains can cause skin damage by irritating the surrounding skin. In chronic wounds, proteases, particularly matrix metallo-proteinases, are thought to actively damage healthy skin through their enzymatic action (Trengrove et al 1996).

Cutting (1999) describes how the stratum corneum initially absorbs fluid, causing swelling. Further saturation reduces barrier function, leading to skin breakdown.

Exudate can be controlled by using absorbent dressing materials (e.g. **alginates** and hydrophilic foams), by frequent dressing changes or by using a barrier cream (Baranoski & Ayello 2004).

Excessive granulation tissue (proud flesh)

Granulation tissue can be produced in excessive amounts and rise above the level of the skin. Epithelium will not cover this tissue and intervention is required to flatten the wound surface and so facilitate re-epithelialization (Harris & Rolstad 1993). Several treatments are available including the application of silver nitrate sticks (75%) and corticosteroid cream. The use of foam dressings has been described as an effective method of flattening excessive granulation tissue (Dealey 1999).

MANAGING WOUND INFECTION

Management of wound infection presents nurses with difficult challenges. The number of micro-organisms and their pathogenicity will determine the extent of an infection (Leaper & Harding 2000). In health, host defences often resist all but the most pathogenic organisms but in ill health this ability is diminished (Gardener & Frantz 2004). Infection can cause systemic problems, delay healing and prolong hospital stays (Stotts 2000). Prevention of wound infection related to the physical hospital environment may be achieved by:

- ensuring that adequate space is maintained between the beds of patients. Where insufficient space is available, particularly in an open ward, the wound infection rate increases. NHS Estates (2002) recommend that beds should be at least 3.6 metres apart in order to prevent cross-infection
- reducing the time between admission and operation to a minimum. Using preadmission clinics and day surgery units is one way of achieving this. The longer the patient is in hospital, the greater the chance of colonization by the pathogenic bacteria found in hospital
- only preparing patient's skin in theatre or stop shaving skin altogether. The lowest clean wound infection rate is 0.9% where patients are not shaved pre-operatively, compared with 2.5% when patients are shaved (Dealey 1999)
- reducing time spent operating as much as possible. The prolonging of time spent operating increases the risk of infection in clean wounds (Dealey 1999)
- avoiding contamination at the time of operation. An infection rate of 2–5% is expected in clean, elective operations, compared with 40% in emergency, contaminated surgery (Leaper & Harding 2000)
- avoiding the use of drains as this increases the risk of wound infection (Bale & Leaper 2000). Where drains cannot be avoided and are needed to minimize dead space, evacuate haematoma or fluids; closed disposable suction drains result in less wound infection than an open drainage system (Bale & Leaper 2000)
- using good hand-washing techniques.

Where wound infection has developed, the management of the individual will depend on a number of factors.

Management of patients with MRSA-positive wound swabs

1. General skin care. Screen patients fully (i.e. swab axillae, nose, throat and perineum) and treat with mupirocin ointment 2% topically for 5–7 days only (RCN 2004) or follow trust policy. In addition, applying an antiseptic lotion, containing triclosan or chlorhexidine, may eradicate skin colonization.
2. Follow trust policy. May include application of mupirocin daily to the wound bed. Alternatively, topical antiseptics such as povidone iodine or silver sulphadiazine may be used to eliminate wound colonization (RCN 2004).
3. Swab at weekly intervals following treatment. The patient is considered clear when three consecutive negative swabs have been obtained.
4. Where topical mupirocin is not effective, consider using a short course of rifampicin systemically together with another antibiotic to which the strain is sensitive (Duckworth 1993).
5. Use an isolation unit, ward or side room. Keep the door closed as much as possible, especially during bed making, wound care, suctioning or moving the patient (RCN 2004).

Figure 3.10
A patient 10 days following reduction mammoplasty showing signs of gross wound infection.

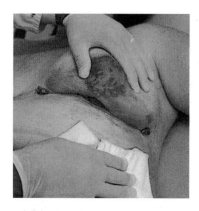

Figure 3.11
Removing the suture to release pus and infected fluid.

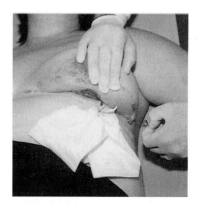

Figure 3.12
The resultant cavity wound.

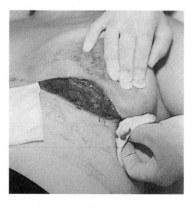

6. Where patients have a serious infection, vancomycin can be administered intravenously.

Surgical wound infection

Surgical wound infection has been defined as one that occurs at the site of surgery within 30 days of surgery or within one year if an implant has been inserted (Stotts 2000). Surgical wound infection can be categorized into superficial, which only involves the skin and subcutaneous tissue of the incision, and deep, which involves the deep soft tissues (Gardener & Frantz 2004).

Figure 3.13
Wound prior to
assessment.

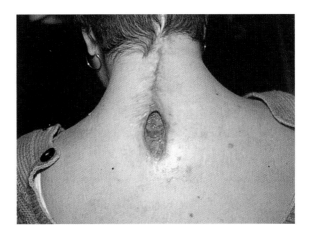

Figure 3.14
Following probing, a large
cavity is detected under
the suture line.

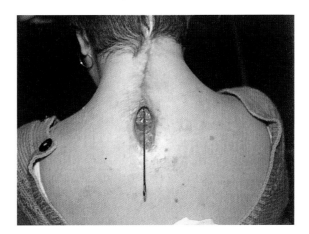

Localized wound infection

Sutured wounds that develop a localized infection often discharge spontaneously, so draining the infection. It may be necessary to remove one or two sutures to facilitate complete drainage (Figures 3.10–3.12). A specimen of pus can be sent for culture and sensitivity if antibiotic therapy is being considered. Once the pus has been drained, a packing material such as an alginate rope can be inserted into the wound to maintain drainage and allow the wound to heal from its depths.

When drainage of the abscess is not complete, surgical incision may be required, especially if the abscess is deep-seated; again, a dressing is used to ensure sound healing from the base of the wound (Figures 3.13, 3.14).

Infection in open granulating wounds

Following assessment and the results of bacteriological culture and sensitivity, it may be appropriate either to treat the patient with systemic antibiotics or to apply local antiseptics to the wound bed to eradicate the pathogen causing the wound infection (Gardener & Frantz 2004).

While a wound infection persists it may be wise to perform more frequent wound cleansing and apply a medicated dressing, in an attempt to reduce the bacterial count at the wound bed (Stotts 2000).

Wound care procedures

There are fundamental principles that need to be adhered to when undertaking wound care procedures (Rolstad et al 2000). These are universal precautions where clean, non-sterile gloves are used to remove a soiled dressing and then discarded and a new pair of gloves used for any further procedures (Stotts 1997).

Cleaning, if required at all, is best carried out by irrigation (see below), as swabbing the wound only results in organisms being redistributed around the wound site (Flanagan 1997). Application of basic principles such as use of gloves, hand washing, wound irrigation and sterile dressings can be adapted both to the hospital patient in a surgical ward with an acute wound and to the patient nursed at home with chronic leg ulcers.

Wearing gloves should never replace scrupulous hand washing but is an essential precaution when the skin is broken, as transmission of blood-borne viruses such as human immunodeficiency virus (HIV) is possible through damaged skin (RCN 2004, Stotts 2000).

When managing patients with chronic wounds, simple bathing or showering is recommended (Flanagan 1997). This is considered to cleanse the wound and the surrounding skin and to offer psychological benefit.

Hand washing

The most effective method of preventing cross-infection is to use a good hand-washing technique. This is the cornerstone of the prevention of the spread of infection. As with the rest of the skin, hands carry bacteria that are permanently resident and which can only be eradicated for a few hours (Boyce & Pittet 2002). However, the skin can also be contaminated with transient pathogenic organisms, especially when hands are wet, rings are worn and skin is damaged, which are picked up and then shed. It is possible to remove these pathogenic organisms by adequate hand washing (Rolstad et al 2000). Although many health-care professionals, nurses included, profess to be knowledgeable about the importance of good hand washing, the spread of hospital-acquired infections such as MRSA is evidence that not enough health workers are practising the technique effectively (Pittet 1999). The thoroughness of the hand washing depends on the task to be done.

- *Social* hand washing is undertaken before and after patient contact, when starting work, finishing work, before meal breaks, after using the lavatory and when visiting other wards and departments. Soap and water are adequate for this purpose.
- *Hygienic* hand washing is undertaken before invasive procedures, after contact with infected patients, after procedures involving high-risk patients and after handling contaminated equipment. An antiseptic hand-washing agent is used.
- *Surgical* hand washing is undertaken in preparation for surgical procedures. A three-minute hand-washing procedure using an antiseptic agent is required.

Basic hand-washing technique

Soap and water are usually adequate but alcohol hand cleanser could be substituted where hands are socially clean (RCN 2004). These guidelines also recommend that in the community where soap and water are not available,

Figure 3.15
Hand-washing technique –
see text for more details
(reproduced with kind
permission from Pittet
1999).

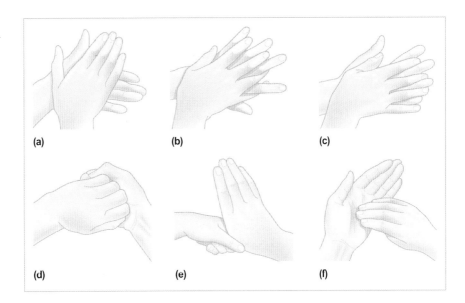

(a)   (b)   (c)

(d)   (e)   (f)

alcohol hand cleanser is useful. All areas of the hands should be cleansed to ensure that they are thoroughly clean.

- Palm to palm
- Right palm over left dorsum and left palm over right dorsum
- Palm to palm with fingers interlaced
- Backs of fingers to opposing palms with fingers interlocked
- Rotational rubbing of right thumb clasped in left palm and vice versa
- Rotational rubbing backwards and forwards with clasped fingers of right hand in palm of left hand and vice versa.

These steps may be difficult to follow. The makers of antiseptic agents have produced pictures of these steps that can be secured over sinks to assist in hand washing (Figure 3.15).

WOUND CLEANSING

Despite the lack of evidence, routine cleansing of wounds is still practised in many areas of wound care (Jones et al 1995, Towler 2001), with nurses unsure of which wound-cleansing procedure to perform (Davies 1999). Indications for cleansing are clear if the underlying principles of wound healing and bacterial **colonization** are understood. The following points should be borne in mind before cleansing procedures are undertaken.

Removal of wound exudate

Normal wound repair requires the bactericidal activity and growth factors present in the inflammatory exudate (Cutting & White 2002). Removal of wound fluid through cleansing and then drying of the wound may only deplete the healing tissue of these vital components and contradicts the principles of moist wound healing (Flanagan 1997).

Elimination of bacteria on the wound surface

It is often believed that the presence of bacteria on a wound bed is harmful and that wound cleansing will eliminate bacteria, so promoting a healthy wound bed and healing. However, research has demonstrated that most granulating wound bed surfaces are colonized with bacteria and that these do not often cause a problem or delay in healing (Stott 2000). It is not possible or even advisable (Gardener & Frantz 2004) to remove all bacteria from the wound surface.

Indications for cleansing

Wounds should only be cleansed to remove excess exudate, slough or necrotic tissue and remnants of old dressing material, all of which can become a focus for infection (Flanagan 1997). However, wounds caused by accidental trauma often contain large amounts of debris and are grossly contaminated and these require thorough cleansing (Towler 2001). Patients with thermal injuries also require wound cleansing because the wound is at greater risk of infection, being no longer colonized with normal flora (Wilson 2000).

Types of cleansing fluid

The use of antiseptic cleansing agents is rarely indicated in routine wound cleansing (Rolstad et al 2000) because the required mechanical cleansing to remove excess debris can be safely achieved using water or saline. In addition, research has demonstrated that antiseptic wound-cleansing agents can damage healthy wound cells, inhibiting their viability and phagocytic activity (Hellewell 1997). Several studies have investigated the effectiveness of normal saline, tap water, distilled water, boiled water and antibacterial solutions not only in lowering bacterial counts but also in reducing infection, though no differences have been detected between these solutions (Griffiths et al 2001).

Method of cleansing

As already described, swabbing a wound with cotton wool or gauze swabs is inadvisable and probably ineffective (Flanagan 1997, Towler 2001). Where large amounts of fluid are required to remove debris, this is best achieved by irrigation (Lawrence 1997). It can be difficult to judge the amount of pressure to use without damaging underlying tissue. There are proprietary saline sprays that can be used to irrigate wound beds (Flanagan 1997, Williams 1996), allowing controlled pressure at around 6.5 psi (Towler 2001). Gentle irrigation for normal cleansing can be achieved with use of a syringe or quill or a jug of warmed saline. When water is used, immersing the wound area in a bowl or bath may be an easy way to remove debris or exudate and less painful to the patient (Figures 3.16, 3.17).

Care must be taken, especially in the hospital environment, that baths, bowls or lifting equipment are cleansed properly between patient use (Towler 2001).

Conclusion

Cleansing of a wound should only be performed when clearly indicated and irrigation with saline or water should in most cases be sufficient. Wounds that are clean, with healthy tissue, do not require cleansing and should be left undisturbed to maintain an optimum environment for healing.

Figure 3.16
Wound cleansing for a
patient with leg
ulceration. A bin liner has
been used to prevent
contamination of the
bucket.

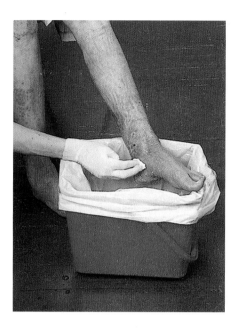

Figure 3.17
Wound irrigation in a
difficult area to treat. This
pressure ulcer was
irrigated with normal
saline using a syringe.

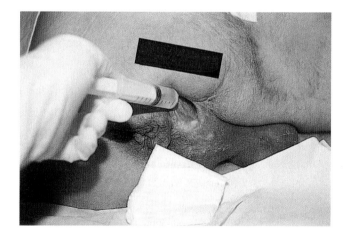

SUMMARY Although wound interventions are becoming more and more sophisticated, the basis of managing any wound successfully is as outlined in this chapter.

Before moving on to the case studies in the rest of the book, ensure that you have understood the following basic principles.

- **The development of dressing materials**
  Moist wound healing
  Range of modern dressings
- **Management of sutured and granulating wounds**
  Signs of infection
  Debridement of devitalized tissue
  Exudate production
- **Prevention of infection**
  Dressing change techniques
  Hand washing
- **Wound cleansing**
  Indications for cleansing
  Methods of cleansing

FURTHER READING

Bale S, Harding K, Leaper D 2000 An introduction to wounds. Emap Healthcare Ltd, London.

Baranoski S, Ayello A E 2004 Wound care essentials: practice principles. Lippincott, Williams and Wilkins, Springhouse, Pennsylvania.

Bryant R A 2000 Acute and chronic wounds: nursing management. Mosby, St Louis, Missouri.

REFERENCES

Ayello A E, Baranoski S, Kerstein M D, Cuddigan J 2004 Wound debridement. In: Wound care essentials: practice principles. Lippincott, Williams and Wilkins, Springhouse, Pennsylvania.

Bale S, Leaper D 2000 Acute wounds. In: An introduction to wounds. Emap Healthcare Ltd, London.

Bale S, Morison M 1997 Wound dressings. In: Morison M, Moffatt C, Bridel-Nixon J, Bale S (eds) A colour guide to the nursing management of chronic wounds. Mosby, London.

Baranoski S, Ayello A E 2004 Wound care essentials: practice principles. Lippincott, Williams and Wilkins, Springhouse, Pennsylvania.

Bergmark M 1967 Vallort och Vitlok: om Folkmedicinens Lakeorter. Natur od Kultur, Stockholm, Sweden.

Boyce J-M, Pittet D 2002 Guidelines for hand hygiene in healthcare settings: Recommendations of the healthcare infection control practices advisory committee and the HICPAC/SHEA/APIC/IDSA hand hygiene task force. Centre for Disease Control, Morbidity and Mortality Weekly Report 17(51): 1–45.

Cutting K F 1999 The causes and prevention of maceration of the skin. Journal of Wound Care 8(4): 200–201.

Cutting K F, White R J 2002 Maceration of the skin and wound bed 1: its nature and causes. Journal of Wound Care 11 (7): 275–278.

Davies C 1999 Cleansing rites and wrongs. Nursing Times 95: 43.

Dealey C 1999 The care of wounds: a guide for nurses. Blackwell Sciences Ltd., Oxford.

Dealey C 2002 Wound healing in Moorish Spain. EWMA Journal 2(1):32–34.

Dealey C 2003 Wound healing in Medieval and Renaissance Italy: was it art or science? EWMA Journal 3(1): 33–35.

Dealey C 2004 The contribution of French surgeons to wound healing in medieval and renaissance Europe. EWMA Journal 1(4): 33–35.

Duckworth G 1993 Diagnosis and management of methicillin-resistant Staphylococcus aureus infection. British Medical Journal 307: 1049–1052.

Dyson M, Young S, Pendle C 1988 Comparison of the effects of moist and dry conditions on dermal repair. Journal of Investigative Dermatology 91(5): 435–439.

Fairbairn K, Grier J, Hunter C, Preece J 2002 A sharp debridement procedure devised by specialist nurses. Journal of Wound Care 11(10): 371–375.

Flanagan M 1997 Wound cleansing. In: Morison M, Moffatt C, Bridel-Nixon J, Bale S (eds) A colour guide to the nursing management of chronic wounds. Mosby, London.

Forrest R D 1982 Early history of wound treatment. Journal of Royal Society of Medicine 75: 198–205.

Gardener S E, Frantz R A 2004 Wound bioburden. In: Wound care essentials: practice principles. Lippincott, Williams and Wilkins, Springhouse, Pennsylvania.

Griffiths R, Fernandez R, Ussia C 2001 Is tap water a safe alternative to normal saline for wound irrigation in the community setting? Journal of Wound Care 10(10): 407–411.

Harris A, Rolstad B S 1993 Hypergranulation tissue: a non-traumatic method of management. In: Harding K G, Cherry G, Turner T D (eds) Proceedings of the Second European Conference on Advances in Wound Management. Macmillan, London.

Hellewell T 1997 A cytotoxicity evaluation of antimicrobial and non-antimicrobial wound cleansers. Wounds 9(1): 15.

Hinman C, Maibach H 1963 Effects of air exposure and occlusion on experimental human skin wounds. Nature 2000: 377–378.

Hunter J 1835 Lectures on the principles of surgery; chapters XII–XIV (notes taken 1786–87). The workings of John Hunter FRS with notes (vol. 1). London, James Palmer, Royal College of England.

Jones V, Bale S, Harding K G 1995 Assessment of wound cleansing. In: Proceedings of the Fourth European Conference on Advances in Wound Management. Macmillan, London.

Lawrence J C 1997 The use of tap water for cleansing traumatic wounds. Journal of Wound Care 6(9): 413.

Leaper D 1986 The wound healing process. In: Turner T D, Schmidt R S, Harding K G (eds) Advances in wound management. John Wiley, Chichester.

Leaper D 2000 History of wounds and the healing process. In: An introduction to wounds. Emap Healthcare Ltd, London.

Leaper D, Harding K 2000 The problem of wound infection. In: An introduction to wounds. Emap Healthcare Ltd, London.

Naylor I L 1999 Ulcer care in the Middle Ages. Journal of Wound Care 8(4): 208–212.

NHS Estates 2002 Infection control in the built environment. Stationery Office, Norwich.

Pittet D 1999 Compliance with handwashing in a teaching hospital. Annals of Internal Medicine 130(2): 126.

Ramundo J, Wells J 2000 Wound debridement. In: Bryant R A (ed) Acute and chronic wounds: nursing management. Mosby, St Louis, Missouri.

Rhodes P 1986 An outline history of medicine. Butterworths, London.

Rolstad B S, Ovington L, Harris A 2000 Principles of wound management. In: Bryant R A (ed) Acute and chronic wounds: nursing management. Mosby, St Louis, Missouri.

Royal College of Nursing (RCN) 2004 Methicillin resistant Staphylococcus aureus (MRSA): guidance for nursing staff. Royal College of Nursing, London: www.rcn.org.uk.

Stotts N A 1997 Sterile versus clean technique in postoperative wound care of patients with open surgical wounds: a pilot study. Journal of Ostomy Continence Nursing 24: 10.

Stotts N A 2000 Wound infection: diagnosis and management. In: Bryant R A (ed) Acute and chronic wounds: nursing management. Mosby, St Louis, Missouri.

Towler J 2001 Cleansing traumatic wounds with swabs, water or saline. Journal of Wound Care 10(6): 231–234.

Trengrove N, Langton S R, Stacey M C 1996 Biochemical analysis of wound fluid from non-healing and healing chronic leg ulcers. Wound Repair and Regeneration 4: 234–239.

Turner T D 1985 Semiocclusive and occlusive dressings. In: Ryan T J (ed) An environment for healing: the role of occlusion. Royal Society of Medicine Congress and Symposium Series 8. Royal Society of Medicine Press, London.

Williams C 1996 Irriclens: a sterile wound cleanser in an aerosol can. British Journal of Nursing 5(16): 1008–1010.

Wilson R 2000 Massive tissue loss: burns. In: Bryant R A (ed) Acute and chronic wounds: nursing management. Mosby, St Louis, Missouri.

Winter G D 1962 Formation of the scab and rate of epithelialisation of superficial wounds in the skin of the young domestic pig. Nature 193: 293–294.

CHAPTER

Wound care in the baby and young child

4

KEY ISSUES   This is the first of the life-cycle chapters and deals with the neonate, baby and young child.

Clinical Case Studies
Illustrate the aetiology and management of:

- Extravasation injury
- The rare genetic disorder of histiocytosis X
- Purpuric rash of meningococcal meningitis
- Thermal injury caused by a scald
- Traumatic injury caused by a dog bite

Nursing Models
Examples of their application to practice are taken from:

- Riehl's interaction model
- Roy's adaptation model
- Peplau's model

PRACTICE POINTS   As you read through this chapter concentrate on the following:

- the choice of dressings that will alleviate pain and minimize trauma and scarring
- the size and type of dressing suitable for babies and small children
- the ways in which nurses can interact with parents and children to decrease emotional trauma
- the importance of documentation of the wound, however small.

INTRODUCTION   In infants the neonatal period covers the first four weeks of life. When considering the whole life-cycle, the neonatal period is the most hazardous, with mortality being high. The neonatal mortality rate is defined as the number of liveborn infants who die before the age of 28 days per 1000 births in the same year. Although neonatal mortality in the UK has fallen from 9.7/1000 live births in 1976 to 3.6/1000 live births in 2003 and infant mortality from 4.6/1000 to 1.7/1000, the fall in neonatal mortality has been less dramatic since 1990 (DoH 2004). For neonates the first day of life is vital – more neonates die on the first day than during the period from 12 months to 25 years. It follows that caring for neonates and infants with wounds presents nurses with many difficult problems. The most obvious are the smallness and vulnerability of the neonate. In babies born prematurely this is even more pronounced. The main causes of death in children include accidents, congenital abnormalities and cancers (Muscari 2001).

The young child with a wound and wound problems also has special requirements. This is a challenging area of nursing and one in which the creativity and skills of the nurse can be decisive in producing the best possible outcome for the child. The principles of caring for sick children must be considered in conjunction with all the principles of managing patients with wounds as previously discussed (MacQueen 2000).

The principles of managing sick children are dealt with only in relation to issues specific to wound management. Further reading on the management of sick children can be found in paediatric nursing textbooks (see Further Reading).

NURSING INFANTS

When serious illness occurs, the family is often thrown into physical and emotional crisis. With support, many stable families are able to cope, though less stable ones may experience great difficulties (Hazinski 1999). The paediatric ward staff are highly trained in understanding the needs of, and in caring for, the whole family when an infant is admitted to hospital. On admission the immediate goals of the staff include:

- gaining the parents' cooperation and trust
- alleviating anxiety or restoring it to an acceptable level
- preserving the relationships between the parent and infant (MacQueen 2000).

Nurses achieve these goals by:

- explaining all the medical and nursing procedures and enlisting the help and support of parents to promote a feeling of partnership between staff and parents
- encouraging parents to stay with their baby for as long as possible or to visit at any time of the day or night (it is usual for beds or chairs to be provided for parents at the infant's bedside, so that they need not be separated)
- helping the parents to understand that regression often occurs. Boredom can also be a problem for infants. This can be helped by placing interesting toys near the child, by talking and interacting with the child whenever they are close and by allowing siblings and other older children to play with or around the child.

However, hospitalization is being reduced as much as possible and increasing numbers of children are being cared for at home as this is considered to be the best environment (O'Dwyer 2000). Whatever the physical environment a baby or child is nursed in, it is important that they are carefully assessed (Fearon

2000). One of the main principles of nursing sick children is to meet the needs of the child as an individual (Hazinski 1999). This involves:

- recognizing each child as a unique, developing individual whose best interests must be paramount
- listening to children, attempting to understand their perspectives, opinions and feelings and acknowledging their right to privacy (Kay 2000)
- considering the physical, psychological, social, cultural and spiritual needs of the children and their families (Hazinski 1999)
- respecting the right of children, according to their age and understanding, to appropriate information and informed participation in decisions about their care (Colson 2000).

A child may have a wound for a variety of reasons and can easily misunderstand the nature of the wound, why it is there and how it will heal. The role of the child's family is an important factor in planning the wound care of an individual child (Teare 1997). As health care is shared with the family, the parents can become actively involved in delivering wound care to their child. Although it is important to recognize that not all parents will want to become actively involved, the majority can feel happy and comfortable about delivering basic wound care to their child. In this situation the nurse provides the education and support which enables parents to learn the necessary skills.

Children feel more confident when their parents provide as much of their wound care as possible. Children also need little encouragement to take part, often removing surgical tape and dressings and cleansing their own wounds (Teare 1997). The physical surroundings in hospital make a huge difference to the attitude of the child. Children's wards, accident and emergency departments and haematology units, for example, usually provide facilities separate from those of adults that are appropriate to the needs of children.

Pain Assessment of a child's pain and the subsequent effective management of that pain can be extremely difficult (Butler 2000). In children acute pain can result in restlessness and agitation, tachycardia, hypertension, pupil dilation, crying and being difficult to comfort.

Historical attitudes to children's experiences of pain are interesting. Although much research had been undertaken on pain in the adult, it was not until the 1970s that pain was considered to be an important issue in paediatrics (Hazinski 1999).

Children may have difficulties in expressing and communicating to others that they are experiencing pain and also in describing what sort of pain they have (Llewellyn 1994). With careful observation nurses and parents can help assess a child's pain in three ways:

- by listening carefully to the child; young children may use a variety of different phrases to express that they are in pain, whereas older children can be quite specific
- by observing changes in the child's behaviour (the parent may report such changes)
- the child may show physiological signs of pain such as increased pulse rate, raised blood pressure and respiratory rate.

To help children express their level of pain, visual scales have been developed to assess pain and a variety of pharmacological and psychological methods of relieving pain (Butler 2000, Hazinski 1999).

Wound management, including dressing changes, need not be associated with pain or discomfort. The nurse's skill in assessing the child with a wound should ensure that the most appropriate wound treatment and dressing are chosen to minimize trauma at dressing changes (Teare 1997).

Dressings suitable for children

In hospital the ward nurse can support and encourage the parents to learn to care for the child's wound. Once the child is home the community nurse is able to continue this support. The child may wish to return to school, nursery or more normal activity before the wound is completely healed. A wide range of dressing materials is available to meet the needs of children with different wound types and problems (Bale & Jones 1996). The choice of dressing and wound care needs to be a joint decision between the child, parents and nurse. Certain dressing materials are particularly suitable for children, especially those that provide an occlusive or semiocclusive environment. As discussed in Chapter 3, these materials include semipermeable films and hydrocolloids that are self-adherent and isolate the wound from the outside environment. The child is thus able to play and bathe without the parents having to worry about the wound getting dirty or wet. For deeper, cavity wounds semipermeable films can be used to hold other dressing materials in place, for example alginates, gels and foams.

Caution is needed when applying topical agents to large areas in the neonate, as absorption (for example, of calcium from alginates) may interfere with their delicate electrolyte balance. The majority of modern dressing materials are soft, conformable and comfortable and come in a wide range of sizes so that small children are well catered for.

Wound cleansing and dressing application

It can be extremely difficult to perform a strict aseptic technique on a baby or small child. Small children are easily distracted and get bored and also may be frightened by a dressing pack and equipment. Even using gloves can cause some children great distress. Hands cleansed with gel can be used for wound dressing and dressing changes either by a parent or the nurse (Kay 2000). As an alternative, the use of a showerhead or bowl of water may provide a less frightening alternative to wound irrigation with a syringe and quill (Bale & Jones 1996, Teare 1997). As with adults, wound cleansing and dressing changes should only be carried out when indicated. Such indications include the presence of devitalized tissue, infection or excess exudate production. Unnecessary repeated wound cleansing and dressing changes will only traumatize newly forming tissue.

Returning to normal activity

Wound therapies and dressing should permit the child to have as near normal day-to-day activities as possible. To facilitate this the nurse may choose dressing materials that are not bulky or use items of clothing to hold dressings in place. In small babies, napkins can be used to hold dressings in the perineal area in place. Children may also pull or fiddle with their dressings and it may be necessary to apply a pad and bandage over the top to prevent this.

EXTRAVASATION INJURY

Extravasation injuries may occur as a consequence of the difficulty of giving intravenous fluids to small children. Case study 4.1 describes a typical problem.

Case study 4.1

Extravasation injury

Ten-day-old Samantha Marks was born at 40 weeks' gestation and was a well-developed full-term neonate. Following a normal delivery, Samantha was progressing well until five days after delivery she became restless and irritable, refusing to feed, and was found to be pyrexic (38°C). Microbiological examination revealed that she had a Gram-negative septicaemia that was immediately treated with a course of intravenous antibiotics, via an infusion that was sited in her left foot.

During infusion the cannula became dislodged and a large amount of antibiotic solution invaded the subcutaneous tissue of her foot. The infusion was resited in the right foot but the damage to the left foot resulted in an area of inflamed tissue that extended over the whole of the dorsal area.

Initially treated with dry dressing by the paediatric nurses, within three days the inflamed area became necrotic and sloughy, exuding large amounts of exudate, and inflammation began to spread up Samantha's leg. The area was obviously very painful when touched and, although her general condition was now improving, the wound was causing Samantha and her parents great distress (Figure 4.1).

Figure 4.1
Extravasation injury.

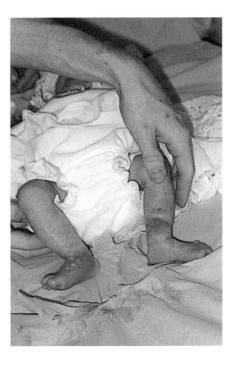

Aetiology
In neonates an infusion may be sited in the scalp or foot as cannulation in the cubital fossae or hands is technically difficult (Mohammed 2000). During illness some infants will require fluids to be given intravenously. Infants have a higher fluid requirement in proportion to their surface area than adults and during illness, the basal metabolic rate can significantly increase. In infants the kidneys are immature and so fluid intake must be closely monitored (Hazinski 1999).

Extravasation injuries are often the result of intravenous solutions leaking into the surrounding tissue. Infiltration of fluid may result in scarring or amputation with fatal consequences (Young 1995). A higher percentage of injuries occur when infusions are sited in lower limbs and, in some situations, damage occurs to the nerves and tendons, with ensuing tissue death and necrosis.

Management
Should extravasation occur, the infusion must be stopped immediately, the cannula removed, the doctor advised and the pharmacist contacted to advise on the potential toxicity of the infused substance. Prevention of this type of tissue injury can be best achieved by frequent observation of the infusion site. It is therefore advisable to secure cannulae with a semipermeable film dressing rather than bandage. Nothing replaces careful observation of these sites by the nurse, as even intravenous delivery pumps are not considered reliable in detecting extravasation. Management of the resulting injury is essential as extensive tissue death could result in further damage with disastrous consequences.

The commonest method of management is the use of a sterile polythene bag containing a hydrogel (Bale & Jones 1996) or hydrogel covered with film. In extreme cases debridement, grafting and secondary reconstruction may be necessary so it is important that nurses monitor extravasation sites by measuring and documenting the position of the injury, the amount and type of wound tissue (e.g. necrotic, sloughy or granulating) and the extent and spread of erythema.

Nursing model for Samantha

When dealing with such a young infant, the nurse's role will depend largely on interaction with Samantha's parents but the type of nursing care given to Samantha's wound could have a profound effect on the rest of her life. The damage has been done but further deterioration of the wound could result in her losing the use of her foot or even the foot itself.

When choosing a model for Samantha consider the following priorities of care:

- the *trauma* to the parents of having their new baby become so ill in a short space of time
- their *understanding* of the situation: do they know what has caused the injury to Samantha's foot?
- do they realize the potential problems that could arise from *mismanagement* of the wound?
- Samantha still has to *recover* fully from her septicaemia
- Samantha is experiencing *pain* when her foot is handled; this may discourage her parents from picking her up and cuddling her
- do the nurses understand the *legal* implications of this baby's care?

Table 4.1
Use of the FANCAP mnemonic to plan Samantha's care

	Physiological	**Psychological**	**Sociological**
Fluids	Needs to maintain necessary fluid intake orally and intravenously	Parents may not wish further IV fluids to be given because of extravasation	
Aeration	Necrotic tissue to be removed to facilitate healing of wound	Parents need to understand *how* and *why* necrotic tissue is removed	
Nutrition	Needs bottle feeds to be introduced	Parents frightened to feed baby owing to illness	Mother unsure how to feed baby
Communication	Doctors and nurses need to explain implications of injury Documentation essential	Parents frightened or angry at hospital, doctors and nurses as to why this injury has occurred	Parents may consider legal action against hospital
Activity	Baby needs to be cuddled and handled normally Left foot needs to regain normal movement		Parents need to understand importance of bonding
Pain	Dressings chosen that minimize pain on removal Do not restrict movement of foot	Nurses and parents frightened to change dressings if causing Samantha distress and pain	

Look at the emphasized points: *trauma, understanding, mismanagement, recover, pain* and *legal*. All these points focus on the parents', nurse's and baby's *perceptions* of the situation. The type of environment in which the baby is nursed will greatly affect the parents' perception of this situation. An environment full of equipment and staff busying themselves with the baby may alienate the parents and they will feel they are not being told everything. Although in Samantha's case her physiological care is important, the nurse must concentrate also on the psychological and sociological parameters to help the parents deal with their baby's illness. Riehl's interaction model addresses these issues (Riehl-Sisca 1989) and she advocates the use of the FANCAP system (Fluids, Aeration, Nutrition, Communication, Activity and Pain) developed by Abbey (1980) to assess patients' needs. This can be applied to Samantha's needs as shown in Table 4.1.

PRACTICE POINTS
- Some of the problems have been highlighted; can you identify any others?
- The management of the wound can be achieved with the use of a hydrogel as previously outlined, which can be covered by using either a sterile plastic bag or film dressings. The bag method is preferable because the wounds are visible and pain is minimized as there is no trauma when removal takes place, as might occur with overzealous use of films.
- This situation should be organized by an experienced paediatric team leader, as it is essential that parents and nurses are kept informed of the implications of this type of injury.

HISTIOCYTOSIS X *Histiocytosis X is a rare congenital disorder. The case described in Case study 4.2 illustrates the problems of managing perineal wounds in babies.*

Case study 4.2

Histiocytosis

Simon James had been a healthy, normal baby until he was five months old, when he developed a generalized rash. This was initially diagnosed as eczema and treated by his general practitioner with emollients and steroid creams, both of which had little effect.

He was referred to a dermatologist, who admitted him to hospital for further investigation and treatment. Skin biopsies of the rash revealed a diagnosis of Langerhans' cell histiocytosis X. Within five days of admission Simon's condition deteriorated and he required artificial ventilation owing to respiratory distress. In conjunction with his general deterioration, Simon's rash had broken down and ulcerated, with large areas of necrotic eschar covering his abdomen and perineum (Figure 4.2). The perineal area was also contaminated with urine and faeces and the staff of the paediatric intensive care unit were having trouble keeping a dressing on such a small infant.

Simon's mother was a single parent and lived in poor social circumstances. She had limited understanding of the severity of her son's condition and found it distressing to see his wound dressings being changed, as often they would stick to the skin, causing Simon to cry.

Aetiology

Congenital abnormalities

Anatomical defects present at birth are classified as congenital abnormalities. This includes, but is not limited to, hereditary disorders.

Congenital abnormalities occur for several reasons. They can be inherited, caused by an embryological defect or can be idiopathic. About 1 in 100 babies is born with a severe malformation, accounting for 1 in 5 stillbirths and 1 in 10 infant deaths.

Figure 4.2
Simon James with a large necrotic area on the groin and abdomen.

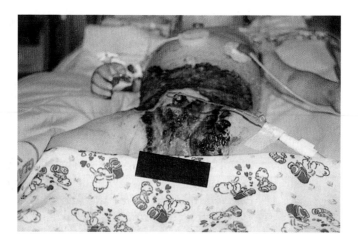

Histiocytosis X

Histiocytosis X is an extremely rare disorder that affects mainly children under the age of two years. The disorder derives its name from the type of body cell involved, the histiocyte (macrophage), with -*osis* meaning increased numbers and X denoting that the cause is unknown.

There are two main types of histiocytosis X; single system and multisystem. In single-system histiocytosis X only one organ in the body is affected, whereas in multisystem disease more than one organ is involved. This disorder is often confused with malignant disease; histiocytosis X is not a type of cancer. The histiocytes do not multiply in situ in an unorganized way but tend to migrate to a site in abnormal numbers or stray outside their normal tissue compartment. Children with histiocytosis X have a deficiency of a certain type of white blood cell, the suppressor lymphocyte (Riggs & Bale 1993).

Prognosis varies. A high incidence of spontaneous remission occurs in single-system disease. Although patients with multisystem disease may spontaneously remit, these children often need treatment. Generally, the younger the child when diagnosed and the more organs involved, the poorer the prognosis. When histiocytosis is diagnosed in older children the disease often runs a more chronic course and may not be life threatening although there is associated morbidity, leaving the child with chronic problems.

Management

Managing a wound in the perineum is a difficult nursing problem. Faecal and urinary contamination in a young infant with no bladder or bowel control is inevitable. Frequent wound hygiene is required to keep the bacterial count as low as possible, in combination with dressings that are easily and quickly changed. Use of a hydrogel together with a hydrocellular dressing may seem an expensive option but several points need to be considered:

- pain and distress are avoided using these dressings
- hydrogels are quickly and easily removed when changing a napkin
- the treatment is effective (Figure 4.3).

Figure 4.3
Simon following wound debridement with hydrogel and hydrocellular dressings. The dressings have been held in place with his napkin.

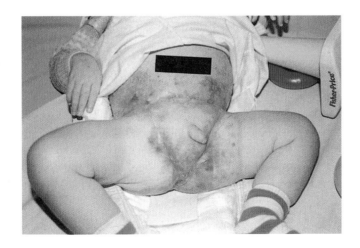

Table 4.2

Use of Roy's adaptation model to assess Simon's care

Life area	Assessment Level 1 – Behaviour	Assessment Level 2 – Stimuli		
		Focal	Contextual	Residual
Physiological nutrition elimination oxygenation regulation	Not taking food orally	Unconscious	Mechanical ventilation	
	No bladder or bowel control	Not yet learnt	Physiological development	
	Unable to breathe spontaneously	Disease process		
	Necrotic wound areas over perineum and abdomen	Disease process		Rash previously undiagnosed
	Dressings not staying in place	Difficult area to dress	Inexperience of staff dealing with wound	
	Wound contamination	Bladder and bowel incontinence	No continence aids in use	
	Infection of wounds	Cross-contamination from staff Immunosuppressed by disease	High-risk hospital area	
Rest and exercise	Normal activity stopped Nursed in frightening environment	Sudden onset of illness	Intensive therapy unit setting	
Self-concept	No familiar surroundings to lessen anxiety		Hospital surroundings	Never been in hospital
	Mother unable to understand severity of condition	Sudden onset of illness	Lack of intellectual skills	
Role function	Mother unable to provide care, loss of mother role	Mother excluded from care	Lack of social skills to cope	
Interdependency	Dependent on staff to provide care	Child too ill, needs specialist staff		No previous experience in hospital
	Mother feels helpless		No support from family, single mother	No previous experience in hospital
	Mother distressed at dressing changes	Not always present when dressings done	Lack of understanding of dressing procedure	No previous hospital experience

Nursing model for Simon

Simon was a previously well infant; both he and his mother now have to *adapt* to the changes in his health status. A model that deals with *loss* of adaptation to ill health is Roy's adaptation model (Roy & Andrews 1999), which can be used to plan Simon's care as shown in Tables 4.2 and 4.3.

Table 4.3

Care plan for Simon

Problem	Goal	Intervention
Unable to breathe spontaneously (A)	Restore oxygenation to normal level	Artificial ventilation
Lack of nutrition (A)	Provide normal nutrition	IV nutrition (check)
Wound contamination from urine (A)	Prevention of urinary incontinence soiling wound	Indwelling catheterization until wound healed
Large amount of necrotic tissue over perineum and abdomen (A)	Removal of necrotic tissue to facilitate healing	Daily application of hydrogel to promote autolysis
Contamination of wound with faeces (A)	Removal of faeces from wound site	Highly absorbent hydrocellular dressing (Allevyn) to remove excess faecal fluid from wound site
Dressings not staying in place	Minimize disturbance of dressing	Secure with baby's nappy over Allevyn sheet
Wound infection (P)	Prevent introduction of infection	Strict asepsis when dressing wound Hand-washing between contacts and when handling soiled napkins
Lack of normal environment (A)	Minimize fear of environment	Staff always to talk, touch and smile with baby Avoid excess use of alarm systems on machines Keep familiar toys and pictures around bed area
Loss of role for mother	Promote mother's involvement	Include mother in care where possible Explain to her why particular treatments are carried out Encourage her to talk to and touch baby
Mother unable to understand severity of condition	Explain in clear terms child's prognosis	Doctors and nurses to use non-medical terms to explain condition Inform mother of changes Do not talk 'over' mother, always with her Involve social worker/health visitor to assess home conditions
Mother anxious at surroundings	Minimize her anxiety level	Encourage mother to voice fears to staff Allow time alone with baby if requested Allow time for her to ask questions
Mother distressed at dressing changes	Ensure pain-free dressing changes	Change dressings daily Soak dressings off if signs of adherence Allow mother to help if desired Explain nature and action of dressing products

(A), actual problem; (P), potential problem.

PRACTICE POINTS

- The emphasis of this care plan is placed on minimizing the trauma of being nursed in a 'high technology' area.
- The mother should be involved in Simon's care but only when and if she desires it.
- Her distress at the dressing changes is possibly the way in which she expresses her general anxiety about his overall condition. However, it is one area of care in which she could be involved, provided she has adequate support and guidance.

INFECTIOUS DISEASES

One of the most serious infectious diseases in small children is meningitis, as described in Case study 4.3.

Case study 4.3

Infectious diseases

Lisa Evans, a previously healthy 11-month-old child, has been ill for the past week with a cold, cough and sore throat.

Her condition deteriorated one evening when she became very hot and began to vomit. Following three episodes of vomiting she became listless and appeared to be losing consciousness. Her mother called the general practitioner who arranged her immediate admission to hospital with suspected meningococcal meningitis.

Following admission, Lisa was transferred to the intensive care unit for intubation and intravenous antibiotic therapy. By the following day she had developed a purpuric rash over her trunk, buttocks and legs and she was diagnosed as having meningococcal septicaemia (Figure 4.4).

Within the next three days the purpuric rash had spread to involve both arms and was blistering, necrotic and wet. Lisa had responded well to her antibiotics and was breathing spontaneously but remained nursed in a high-dependency area off the intensive care unit.

Epidemiology

Although the risk of contracting meningitis is very small, infection rates are highest in children under the age of five, in whom meningococcal infection can cause severe illness very quickly (Heyderman et al 2003, Phillips & Simor 1998). Despite the numerous medical advances that have taken place in paediatrics, the mortality and morbidity rates from meningitis have not decreased. Babies are at higher risk of getting meningitis because they do not have fully developed immune systems and those born earlier than 33 weeks and those weighing less than 2000 g are more at risk (Meningitis Research Foundation 2002). Almost 10% of affected children die and permanent defects affect over 30% of the survivors. The incidence of bacterial meningitis is highest in the first 12 months following birth, with the rates falling as childhood progresses.

Figure 4.4
Purpuric rash of meningococcal meningitis in a seven-year-old child.

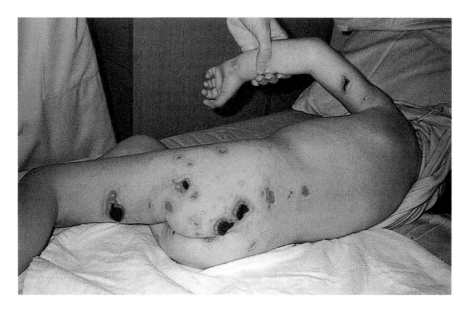

Aetiology   Meningitis is inflammation of the meninges, the membranes covering the brain and spinal cord (Phipps 1998). Bacterial meningitis is an acute, life-threatening infection that requires early diagnosis and appropriate treatment if the patient is to stand the best chance of survival (Spach 2003). There is a decline in the incidence of bacterial meningitis in children, thought to be due to the introduction of immunization programmes since the 1980s (Heyderman et al 2003, Spach 2003). Organisms causing meningitis vary; interestingly, different pathogens affect specific age groups:

- neonate: group B streptococci, coliform bacteria
- 1 month onwards: *Haemophilus influenzae, Neisseria meningitidis, Streptococcus pneumoniae*
- 1–4 years: *Haemophilus influenzae.*

Diagnosis of meningitis is difficult, with symptoms being vague and in the first instance identical to many other, less dangerous, childhood illnesses. Typically the infant will develop a generalized febrile illness with unusual irritability or lethargy (Hazinski 1999). This rapidly develops to include other symptoms such as vomiting and seizures as the infant's condition deteriorates. Nuchal rigidity or a bulging fontanelle occurs in less than 50% of infants and small children (Phillips & Simor 1998). The purpuric rash of meningococcal meningitis is associated with an overwhelming infection with Gram-negative diplococcus or meningococcus, thus causing haemorrhage through toxic damage to the capillaries. Skin damage from this rash can often be so severe that full-thickness skin loss and ulceration result in permanent damage. Other long-term complications include hearing loss, seizures and learning difficulties (Phillips & Simor 1998).
Diagnosis is based on:

- the presence of a non-specific febrile illness
- raised intracranial pressure, clinical signs of which include reduced and declining level of consciousness, extensor hypertonia, cranial nerve palsy, dilated pupils, bradycardia and high blood pressure

- positive blood culture
- lumbar puncture to obtain cerebrospinal fluid, which will demonstrate raised levels of white cells and protein and reduced glucose concentration.

Management

Patient outcome is dependent on early diagnosis and treatment. Third-generation cephalosporins offer a safer and more effective alternative to the previously popular antibiotic regimens of chloramphenicol and penicillins. However, there is an increasing resistance of bacteria to some antibiotics (Phillips & Simor 1998). These infants are best nursed on paediatric intensive care units with aggressive support of cardiovascular function, elective ventilation and measures to reduce raised intracranial pressure. If the infant survives this acute stage of the illness, bacterial toxins can cause other problems such as vascular damage.

Ulceration can be treated with excision and grafting, a process that will hasten healing but will depend on the child's general condition and the availability of plastic surgery. Alternatively, hydrogels, hydrocolloids or silver sulphadiazine creams will soften eschar and debride wounds (Bale & Jones 1996, MacQueen 2000). This may be the easiest option for parent and child for care that continues in the community (Teare 1997). These materials are readily available on prescription at home. Hydrocolloid sheets are occlusive and permit bathing and playing, without risking wound contamination from the outside environment. At this age babies are crawling, rolling and learning to stand; they may also pull at dressings that are not firmly fixed. Difficulty may arise with the use of hydrocolloids as the dressing stays in place for several days at a time, so wound inspection would not be possible on a daily basis. Hydrogels and silver sulphadiazine may need to be used in conjunction with a film dressing to make this a practical option. Again, bathing, playing and crawling around would not disturb the dressings. Frequent wound inspection is possible as the dressing would need to be changed on a daily basis.

Nursing model for Lisa

Lisa's condition is life threatening and although the nurse needs to establish a good relationship with her parents, her first priority will be assessing Lisa's physical condition.

The correct management of the child's wound at this stage may avoid or minimize the scarring that could result from her meningococcal rash. Using Peplau's model, assess Lisa's needs under the SOAP structure (Peplau 1952).

S – Subjective feelings and experiences of the patient or parent, e.g. mother concerned at the large amount of 'black scabs' on wound

O – Objective observation by nurse, e.g. large areas of necrotic tissue preventing wound from healing

A – Formal assessment and identification of problem. Problem statement or goal: necrotic tissue requiring removal

P – Plan of action:
- apply hydrogel to facilitate autolysis
- apply low-adherent dressings

S – Mother anxious that Lisa will not recover from meningitis

O – Vital signs now within normal limits and baby recovering:
- baby breathing spontaneously

Figure 4.5
Baby Lisa showing
wounds healed.

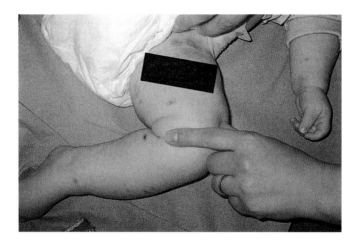

- displays no signs of cerebral irritation
  A – Mother's anxiety level high
  P – Provide mother with information and reassurance of baby's recovery:
- encourage mother to stay with baby
- inform mother of changes in baby's condition
- encourage mother to participate in baby's care.

PRACTICE POINTS
- Observations could also be made concerned with recording the wound size, ensuring wounds do not become macerated and that removal of the dressings is painless for the baby.
- The mother will need advice regarding how long treatment of her baby's wounds may take and how she can help care for Lisa during this period (Figure 4.5).

THERMAL INJURIES

Wounds from burns and scalds in young children are frequently found in nursing practice. An example of an accidental injury of this type is given in Case study 4.4.

Case study 4.4

Thermal injuries

Lucy Llewellyn is just two years old and was admitted to Primrose Ward at 10 a.m. as an emergency. Lucy, the youngest of three children, had gone into the kitchen unsupervised this morning and reached up to the kitchen unit to get her teddy bear. Unfortunately she had not seen the full cup of tea her father had left just on the edge and tipped it over herself, scalding her shoulder, upper arm and chest. Her mother, alerted by Lucy's screams, had the foresight to immediately remove the clothing and run the scalded areas under the tap for 10 minutes, and cover the area with a clean tea towel. The father called an ambulance that took her to the local hospital where Lucy was treated for a deep, partial-thickness injury to her shoulder and upper arm and a superficial partial-thickness injury to her chest. Although these injuries were serious, the mother's quick action had prevented further damage.

Epidemiology

Thermal injuries from flame, burns and scalds are extremely common in young children. In the UK 125 000 children require hospital treatment each year (National Burns Care Review Committee 2001), of whom about 50% have been injured in the kitchen following scalds from hot liquids. Here, hot drinks are involved in about 1265 of severe burns, of which 1100 occur in children under the age of five years. Lawrence and Carson (1994) tracked the increase in kettle scalds since the 1920s and report that a marked increase in this injury is related to the introduction of plastic jug kettles.

Management

Correct and prompt first aid management of burns and scalds can substantially reduce the depth of tissue damage. Immediate immersion in cold water for at least 20 minutes rapidly quenches residual heat and eases pain (Dowsett 2002, McCormack et al 2003). Parents, however, may be distressed at their screaming child, not know how long to apply cold water and be alarmed by seeing skin peel off. It should be stressed that the burn or scald will continue to develop with redness and blistering and appear to enlarge. Seconds are often lost by removal of clothing, which should also be drenched to save time (Mertens et al 1997). The burned area should be wrapped in cling film or a clean plastic bag prior to leaving for the hospital as this protects the area from contamination as well as relieving pain from air exposure (Khot & Polmear 2003).

Thermal injuries are classified according to depth (Phipps 1998).

- *Superficial burn*: presents as erythema or mild erythema and pain. The reddened area blanches with pressure. Occurs following sunburn or flash burn. Heals within 3–7 days with no scarring.
- *Partial-thickness skin loss*: fluid lost from the burn wound either forms blisters under damaged skin or exudate from areas where the outer layers have been lost.
  i) Superficial partial-thickness skin loss: the epidermis and superficial layers of the dermis are destroyed. Hair follicles, sebaceous and sweat glands are, however, spared. From these epithelial structures, migration of cells rapidly occurs to provide an intact surface within 10–21 days. Pain is experienced when the nerve endings of the dermis have not been damaged. The wound usually heals without scarring.
  ii) Deep partial-thickness skin loss: a greater part of the dermis is lost and little of the skin appendages remain. Healing is delayed. Sensation is altered – patient has blunting of pinprick sensation.
- *Full-thickness skin loss*: there are no surviving epithelial elements in full-thickness loss. The burn can only heal by contraction and by migration of existing epithelial cells at the edges of the wound. The wound may look pale and charred and coagulated veins may be visible. No sensation is present on testing.

Nursing the child following injury

On admission to the children's ward an initial assessment of the child will take into account that the child has not been prepared for admission and may be very frightened. As a result the child may be fractious and crying, frightened and clinging to her parents. On admission the nurse will aim to:

- use a calm and friendly approach to the child and family to comfort and reassure the child. The child will be assured that her mother or father will be able to stay with her so that she will not be left alone
- encourage the parents to cuddle and care for the child. Intravenous infusions and other equipment need not prevent parents from maintaining close contact with their child
- explain to the child and parents, using terms they will understand, any procedures that may need to be performed
- be non-judgemental, to reassure the parents that blame is not being apportioned. Some parents may want to talk about the accident and may be obviously distressed. The nurse aims to restore the parents' confidence and self-esteem as they may be feeling inadequate and guilty.

Longer-term aims of nursing care are:

- to help the parents understand that their child may take time in adapting to the new environment and that behavioural disturbances are to be expected (Butler 2000). Their child may become aggressive and difficult or, alternatively, may become quiet and withdrawn. Behavioural regression may take many forms and parents need the reassurance that this is temporary
- to encourage the child to become independent again and restore her self-confidence
- to introduce the child to play leaders, nursery nurses and teachers, where appropriate, to minimize boredom. In addition, televisions, videos and computer games can help to alleviate boredom.

Over a period of time the nurse may be able to take on a health educator role in helping the parents to understand how the accident happened and how it may be prevented in the future. This involves looking at a number of factors contributing to the accident and including the child, the agent involved (e.g. the cup of tea) and the physical and social context in which the accident happened.

Non-accidental injury
In the accident and emergency department parents are likely to be closely questioned on how the accident happened and what action they took subsequently. The child may also be asked what happened although in Lucy's case this would not be admissible as she is shocked and distressed. Staff will always ascertain whether the distribution of injury fits the history given by the parents.

Effects of hypertrophic scarring
Unfortunately the hypertrophic scarring following a burn or scald can be a constant disfiguring reminder to the child of the causative accident. Hypertrophic scars are red, firm and thickened and cause intense itching (see Chapter 1).

Although hypertrophic scarring usually flattens as the scar matures, there is evidence that the use of constant, long-term pressure can prevent its formation (Hazinski 1999). Several preventive and treatment options are available for reducing scarring including silicone sheets, pressure garments, chemical peels and vitamin creams (O'Kane 2002). Pressure garments are popular and are used to apply pressure on the torso and limbs and help realignment of the collagen fibres. These are worn for 24 hours daily and removed only for cleansing or bathing for the first nine months (Pape 1993) for a period of up to two years. Garments will need frequent replacement in the growing child and great care is required to ensure they are comfortable and well fitting. The wearing of such garments can have a profound effect on small children and will affect all sorts of normal activities of a two-year-old, such as swimming and the wearing of dresses.

Success has also been achieved with topical application of silicone gel sheeting, although its mode of action is unclear. The sheeting is cut to size and secured with adhesive tape and needs to be worn for several weeks by day and night (SMTL 2004).

Treatment of burns and scalds

On admission to an accident and emergency department, a thorough history of the accident will be taken from the parents and/or child.

For major burn injuries or deep skin loss around the face and neck, the main concern is maintenance of a clear airway. The percentage size of the burn is calculated using the Lund and Browder chart (Figure 4.6). The child's weight is taken and assessment of fluid requirements calculated. If the burn is over 10% of the body surface pain relief and tetanus toxoid will be given where required, depending on the depth and type of burn injury.

Wound dressings

The burn or scald should be swabbed prior to cleansing, to ascertain the type of bacteria present in the wound. Bacterial colonization of all thermal wounds occurs following injury but generally causes no problems with healing, the greatest risk being cross-contamination between patients (Hazinski 1999). Certain organisms, however, may cause particular problems, especially *Staphylococcus aureus* that can result in toxic shock syndrome.

Cleansing should be performed with saline (see Chapter 2), using irrigation techniques. Dead epithelium and blisters are removed using sterile scissors, with debridement of necrotic material under strict aseptic conditions. Deep dermal burns will require surgical debridement in theatre followed by excision and grafting.

Following cleansing, burns should be covered with a low-adherent dressing.

Films and hydrocolloids will provide moist wound healing and protection for superficial burns with low to moderate levels of exudate (Dowsett 2002). More heavily exuding wounds can be dressed with alginates, foams and hydrofibre dressings. Silver sulphadiazine (Flamazine) is widely used as prophylaxis against *Pseudomonas aeruginosa* infection and is useful on hands (in plastic bags), ears and genital areas (Odense Universitetshospital 2004).

Nursing model for Lucy

There are many issues at stake for Lucy and her family. The nurse on the ward needs to build a strong, trusting relationship with the toddler and her parents. As with Samantha (Case Study 4.1), it is important to look at psychological and sociological aspects, as well as physiological care for Lucy and her parents. Riehl's model is therefore a useful framework for the initial assessment. Look at

Figure 4.6
Lund and Browder chart
(reproduced by kind
permission of Smith &
Nephew Pharmaceuticals).

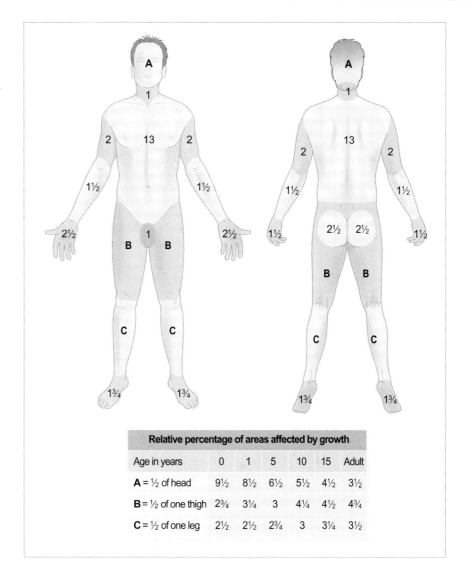

Relative percentage of areas affected by growth						
Age in years	0	1	5	10	15	Adult
A = ½ of head	9½	8½	6½	5½	4½	3½
B = ½ of one thigh	2¾	3¼	3	4¼	4½	4¾
C = ½ of one leg	2½	2½	2¾	3	3¼	3½

the problems identified below and consider how you can help child and parents.
Look at the situation from the parents' and child's points of view.

Physiological (A actual, P potential)
◼ Pain due to burn injury (A)
◼ Risk of infection in wound site (P)
◼ Hypertrophic scarring following wound healing (P)
◼ Dressings adhering to wound causing painful dressing change (P)
◼ Child not wanting nurses to change the dressings (P).

Psychological
◼ Parents, particularly father, feeling guilty about accident (A)
◼ Child not understanding what has happened to her (A)

■ Repeated questioning in accident and emergency department and ward reinforcing feelings of guilt (P).

Sociological
■ Child suddenly put in unfamiliar surroundings owing to emergency admission (A)
■ Lack of parental knowledge with regard to prevention of further accidents (A)
■ Parents separated from other children (A)
■ Parents labelled by ward staff as uncaring and careless (P)
■ Child at risk of non-accidental injury (A).

PRACTICE POINTS

■ There are many psychological factors influencing the parents but the child may have psychological effects in the long term, so this should be considered now.
■ This case highlights the need for the specialist skills of trained paediatric nurses when dealing with traumatic injuries in infants. How the care is planned will depend on the experience of the nurse. Inexperienced practitioners may not even identify some of these problems and may not be equipped to provide the required management.
■ Think of the specific skills that a nurse requires to deal with this case.

ANIMAL BITE WOUNDS

Facial wounds in children are commonly caused by bites from animals (usually dogs). Look at the example in Case study 4.5.

Case study 4.5

Injury from dog bite

Sister Mathews is the practice nurse working in a general practice surgery serving a council estate in a large city. One morning Sally Arnold, an eight-year-old child, was brought in screaming and hysterical by her mother, with her face covered in blood. When the nurse had calmed both mother and child she elicited that the child had been playing with their pet mongrel dog that had suddenly jumped up and bitten her cheek.

Sister Mathews irrigated the wound with copious amounts of saline and examined the size and shape of the affected area. Sally had sustained a single laceration above her left cheekbone that measured 1.3 cm in breadth and 0.5 cm in depth. The initial treatment was closure of the wound with sterile adhesive strips while waiting for the doctor to examine the child.

The doctor, who had only had limited experience with suturing facial wounds, arranged for mother and child to go to the city hospital's accident and emergency department. A plastic surgeon examined the wound and, having excluded damage to the underlying tissues, the wound edges were carefully brought together using paper skin closure strips. The child was prescribed a course of penicillin elixir and asked to return to the hospital in seven days.

Aetiology　Animal bites are a common cause of facial injury. In most Western countries 90% are caused by dog bites and 50–75% affect children (Bernardo et al 2000, Kriesfeld & Bordeaux 1998, Sacks et al 1996). In children facial wounds are involved in around 80% of such injuries (Weiss et al 2004). As an added hazard, animal bites carry the risk of diseases such as tetanus and rabies, although these are less common than infections caused by micro-organisms of the normal flora of the animal's mouth and throat.

Management　Bites are best treated within the first 12–24 hours. Prophylactic broad-spectrum antibiotics are advised in high-risk patients. Skin closure is best achieved using adhesive strips and fine biocompatible sutures (Al-Khaleeb & Shepherd 1995). Where sutures are used, early removal is recommended to help prevent scarring. In facial injuries a plastic surgeon is often consulted prior to attempting suturing to ensure that the best cosmetic effect is obtained. Areas that warrant special attention include the following.

- The lip: repair of lip lacerations needs to be performed with respect to the vermilion border so that puckering is prevented.
- The eyelids: repair of injuries to the area surrounding the eye can take place only after the ophthalmologist has examined the eye.
- Haematomas need to be carefully evacuated prior to wound closure.
- Damage to bone, ducts, blood vessels and nerves should be repaired prior to wound closure.
- Extensive tissue loss: depending on the site and extent of the injury, free grafts, pedicle grafts, flaps and tissue expansion can be used.

For at least the first three months following facial injury, the parents are advised to avoid exposure of the child's face to direct sunlight and prolonged soaking of the skin in water.

Nursing model of care for Sally

Before assessing this child's need, look at the previous section. Can you answer the following questions?

- Why was it necessary to irrigate the wound with copious amounts of saline?
- What other information should the sister obtain about the circumstances of the accident?
- What course of action should the nurse take with regard to the dog?
- Why was the doctor reluctant to suture the wound?
- Why did the child require other management, e.g. antibiotics and/or tetanus vaccine?

PRACTICE POINTS
- You should be able to answer the above questions and include them in your plan of care. If you cannot answer, re-read the previous chapter on management of traumatic wounds.
- Once you have obtained the relevant information, what type of model could you use? See if you can write out a detailed plan including all the management issues raised.

SUMMARY

This chapter has dealt mainly with wounds that have a traumatic aetiology – the most common type of children's wound that nurses have to treat. In this age group it can be seen that direct management of the traumatic wound can often appear straightforward.

Challenges here concern the psychological and sociological traumas surrounding wound care in babies and infants. The models that have been chosen to assess the care in each of the case studies have largely concentrated on these important areas and are not easy options on busy paediatric units. They do, hopefully, encourage the practitioner to think about such issues as:

- communication skills – with child, parents and team members
- legal and moral aspects of care – documentation, non-disclosure of information, choice of treatments
- organizational skills – planned management of care
- dressing choices – alleviation of painful dressing changes, minimization of scarring.

FURTHER READING

Department of Health 2004 PRODIGY guidance – burns and scalds. Department of Health (2004) Infant mortality rates 1976–2003. Available online at: www.statistics.gov.uk. Accessed 24.08.04.

Huband S, Trigg E 2000 Practices in children's nursing. Churchill Livingstone, Edinburgh.

Lawrence J C, Cason C 1994 Kettle scalds. Journal of Wound Care 3(6): 289–292.

REFERENCES

Abbey J 1980 The FANCAP assessment scheme. In: Riehl J P, Roy C (eds) Conceptual models for nursing practice. Appleton-Century-Crofts, New York.

Al-Khaleeb T, Shepherd J P 1995 The management and repair of wounds of the face. Journal of Wound Care 4(8): 359–362.

Bale S, Jones V 1996 The care of children with wounds. Journal of Wound Care 5(4): 177–180.

Bernardo L M Gradner M J, O'Connor J, Amon N 2000 Dog bites in children treated in a pediatric emergency department. Journal of Society of Pediatric Nurses 5 (2): 87–95.

Butler N R 2000 Perinatal problems. In: Huband S, Trigg E (eds) Practices in children's nursing. Churchill Livingstone, Edinburgh.

Colson J 2000 Concepts. In: Huband S, Trigg E (eds) Practices in children's nursing. Churchill Livingstone, Edinburgh.

Department of Health 2004 Infant mortality rates 1976–2003. Available online at: www.statistics.gov.uk. Accessed 24.08.04.

Dowsett C 2002 The assessment and management of burns. British Journal of Community Nursing 7 (5): 230–239.

Fearon J 2000 Assessment. In: Huband S, Trigg E (eds) Practices in children's nursing. Churchill Livingstone, Edinburgh.

Hazinski M F 1999 Manual of pediatric critical care. Mosby, St Louis, Missouri.

Hederman R S, Lambert H P, O'Sullivan I, Stuart J M, Taylor B L, Wall R A 2003 Early management of suspected bacterial meningitis and meningococcal septaemia in Adults. Journal of Hospital Infection 46: 75–77.

Kay J 2000 Hygiene. In: Huband S, Trigg E (eds) Practices in children's nursing. Churchill Livingstone, Edinburgh.

Khot A, Polmear A 2003 Surgical problems. In: Practical general practice: guidelines for effective clinical management. Butterworth-Heinemann, Edinburgh.

Kriesfeld R, Bordeaux S 1998 Injury resulting from dog bites. Available online at: www.nisu.flinders.edu.au. Accessed 20.08.04.

Lawrence J C, Carson C 1994 Kettle scalds. Journal of Wound Care 3(6): 289–292.

Llewellyn N 1994 Pain assessment and the use of morphine. Paediatric Nursing 6(1): 25–30.

MacQueen S 2000 Wound care. In: Huband S, Trigg E (eds) Practices in children's nursing. Churchill Livingstone, Edinburgh.

McCormack A, La Hei E R, Martin H C 2003 First-aid management of minor burns in children: a prospective study of children presenting to the Children's Hospital at Westmead, Sydney. Medical Journal of Australia 178 (1): 31–33.

Meningitis Research Foundation 2002 Meningococcal disease. Available online at: www.meningitis.org. Accessed 20.08.04.

Mertens D M, Jenkins M, Warden G 1997 Outpatient burns management. Nursing Clinics of North America 32 (2): 343–364.

Mohammed T A 2000 Venepuncture and cannulation. In: Huband S, Trigg E (eds) Practices in children's nursing. Churchill Livingstone, Edinburgh.

Muscari M E 2001 Pediatric nursing overview. In: Pediatric nursing. Lippincott, Philadelphia.

National Burns Care Review Committee 2001 National burn care review. British Association of Plastic Surgeons. Available online at: www.baps.co.uk.

Odense Universitetshospital 2004 Available online at: www.ouh.dk/wm139946. Accessed 20.08.04.

O'Dwyer J 2000 Introduction to community. In: Huband S, Trigg E (eds) Practices in children's nursing. Churchill Livingstone, Edinburgh.

O'Kane S 2002 Wound remodelling and scarring. Journal of Wound Care 11(8): 296–299.

Pape S A 1993 The management of scars. Journal of Wound Care 2(6): 354–360.

Peplau H 1952 Interpersonal relations in nursing. G P Putman, New York.

Phillips E J, Simor A E 1998 Bacterial meningitis in children and adults. Postgraduate Medicine 103(3): 116–129.

Phipps A 1998 Evidence based management of patients with burns. Journal of Wound Care 7 (6): 299–302.

Riehl-Sisca J P 1989 The Riehl interaction model. In: Riehl-Sisca J P (ed) Conceptual models for nursing practice, 3rd edn. Appleton and Lange, Norwalk, Connecticut.

Riggs R L, Bale S 1993 Management of necrotic wounds as a complication of histiocytosis X. Journal of Wound Care 2(5): 260–261.

Roy C, Andrews H 1999 The Roy adaptation model, 2nd edn. Appleton and Lange, Stamford, Connecticut.

Sacks J, Kresnow M, Houston B 1996 Dog bites: how big a problem? Injury Prevention 2: 52–54.

SMTL 2004 SMTL datacard for dressing silicone sheet. Available online at: www.dressings.org. Accessed 20.08.04.

Spach D H 2003 New issues in bacterial meningitis in adults. Postgraduate Medicine 114 (5): 65–74.

Teare J 1997 A home care team in paediatric wound care. Journal of Wound Care 6(6): 295–296.

Weiss H B, Friedman D I, Coben J H 2004 Incidence of dog bite injuries treated in emergency departments. Available online at: www.dogexpert.com. Accessed 20.08.04.

Young T 1995 Wound healing in neonates. Journal of Wound Care 4(6): 285–288.

Wound care in teenagers

KEY ISSUES   This chapter outlines the most common wound problems encountered by the teenager.

Clinical Case Studies
Aetiology and management of:

- A young boy sustaining chemical burns caused by battery acid
- Pressure sore in a young girl with spina bifida
- Traumatic injuries due to a road traffic accident

Nursing Models
Examples of their application to practice are taken from:

- Roper's activities of living model
- Orem's model
- Roy's adaptation model

PRACTICE POINTS   As you read through this chapter concentrate on the following.

- inadequate wound management that may affect the rest of the teenager's life
- aspects of privacy, body image and personal identity important to a teenager
- emotional effects that injury may have on the teenager
- devastating effect of disablement or disfigurement on the rest of the teenager's life.

INTRODUCTION   Of all the phases of the life-cycle, adolescence is undoubtedly one of the most difficult. During the adolescent period the individual changes from a child into an adult and strives to achieve social and emotional maturity. The duration of adolescence and the age at which it occurs is difficult to determine, as each individual varies. Adolescence has been defined as a phase of physiologic, physical and psychological change through which an individual progresses to reach maturity (Hazinski 1999, Wheal 1999). Body image issues dominate as peers set standards for appearance and behaviour and peer group pressure is strong. Being accepted by peers is a fundamental issue for youths and at this age individuals may set out to impress others by acting irresponsibly and taking unnecessary risks. Concerns about illness focus on changes in physical appearance that may not be deemed acceptable by peers.

Common behavioural traits exhibited by adolescents include mood swings, rebellion, periodic regression, self-preoccupation and antagonism. Coming to terms with the adult world can be an extremely traumatic time for the young individual. Illness and hospitalization of adolescents can be difficult when often their physical needs take precedence over their emotional needs. Health professionals, including nurses, need to be very aware of the needs and rights of teenagers, especially when considering their independence, privacy and social needs (Hazinski 1999, Taylor et al 1999). Adolescent wards are usually available where teenagers are cared for in specialised units designed to meet their specific needs. Such needs include body image and personal identity issues, independence (social and financial) from parents and help in communicating and developing social skills (Wheal 1999).

Specific problems for adolescents being treated in hospital (Taylor et al 1999) include:

- lack of privacy
- problems associated with change of body image and loss of self-worth
- anxiety related to hospitalization
- regression
- restriction of normal physical activities
- fear of death in the seriously ill
- loss of independence.

The adolescent period is one in which accidental and traumatic injuries are common and both mortality and morbidity rates are high. Wounds frequently result from such injuries. Children and young people from lower social classes IV and V are twice as likely to be the victims of accidents, which cause 50% of deaths in 1–19 year olds, as those from social classes I–III (Page 2002). Overall, compared with younger children, adolescents between 15 and 19 years had a much higher mortality rate of 70 per 100 000 in 1999 (Childstats 2004). Injury, which includes homicide, suicide and unintentional injuries, continues to account for over three out of four deaths among adolescents. Motor traffic-related injuries accounted for 37% of deaths in this age group in 1999, and the motor traffic-related death rate for males was nearly twice that for females (Childstats 2004).

After injuries, leading causes of death for adolescents include cancer, heart disease and birth defects.

CHEMICAL BURNS

Case study 5.1 illustrates the case of a schoolboy injured in an industrial accident with corrosive materials.

Case study 5.1

Chemical burns

David Oskim, a 17-year-old schoolboy, has always had a keen interest in cars and car maintenance. Last month he secured a Saturday job in the local garage as a trainee mechanic. He was particularly pleased as his father had just bought him a car and he was having driving lessons.

The garage owner was pleased to take David on because of his enthusiasm but also because he only needed to pay him a small amount of money. A hard-working, conscientious man, he had little time to give David a proper induction and assumed David was aware of the usual hazards of working in this environment.

One Saturday David was working on an engine that required him to remove and drain the battery. While lifting the battery out of its casing, David let it slip and tipped battery acid over his forearm. The owner, who had not experienced this type of accident before, immediately led David to the washbasin, plunged his arm and hand in a basin of cold water and removed the sleeve of his overall. While telephoning for an ambulance, he told David to keep his arm under the tap. On arrival at the accident and emergency department David was shocked and in a great deal of pain, having sustained a superficial partial-thickness burn to his forearm.

Aetiology

Industrial accidents continue to be part of everyday working life. Fatal accidents have risen from 220 per annum in 1999 to 251 in 2002 with an additional rise in major accidents of 28 154 in 2001 to 28 940 in 2002 (Health and Safety Executive 2004). From a workforce of more than 800 000 in the West Midlands, an average of 55 men per annum are seriously burnt (Lawrence 1990).

The level of first aid these workers receive will greatly affect their prognosis and degree of injury. In a study of first aid received undertaken by Petch and Cason (1993), of the 18 patients admitted to the burns unit as a result of industrial accidents, only seven had received satisfactory first aid while eight had received none at all (Table 5.1).

Table 5.1
First aid received by a selection of patients admitted to the burns unit (reproduced with kind permission from Petch & Cason 1993)

Patient group	First aid received		
	Satisfactory	**Unsatisfactory**	**None**
Children	15	3	6
Adults at home	9	3	10
Industrial cases	7	3	8
Other cases not in or around the home	2	3	2
Total	33	12	26

Figure 5.1
Chemical burn sustained following contact with cement (reproduced by kind permission of Jan Olsen, Burns Unit, Morriston Hospital, Swansea).

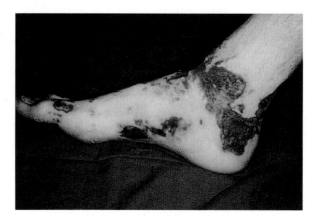

Management

The rapid removal of corrosive chemicals from the skin is an urgent first aid requirement. Highly acid and alkaline substances are readily absorbed into the tissues, causing rapid burning to the affected area (Figure 5.1). Irrigation of the burnt area with copious quantities of water should normally be commenced as soon as possible, with some exceptions. Any clothing in contact with the injured area should be cut away and the skin irrigation continued until an ambulance arrives or en route to the accident and emergency department (Mertens et al 1997). Full details of the nature and composition of the corrosive chemical causing the burn will be needed by the hospital, so every attempt should be made to identify the substance. Some chemicals have specific antidotes that can be given in the accident and emergency department. It is important to note that not all chemical burns should be irrigated with water. Substances containing metallic sodium, potassium and lithium should not be irrigated with water (Dowsett 2002, McCormack et al 2003).

In hospital an assessment of the degree and extent of the burns will be made. The Lund and Browder chart (see Figure 4.6) is now considered to be a more effective method of assessing extent of burns injuries than the 'rule of nine' (Hazinski 1999).

The depth of burn should be assessed and recorded. This can be done by estimating the loss of epidermis, dermis and appendages (see Chapter 4).

Treatment of small burns may be carried out in the accident and emergency department without the need to admit the young person. Removal of dirt and devitalized tissue is essential. Where surgical debridement is needed to remove devitalized tissue, the hospital stay may be only a few days. The use of modern wound dressings for full-thickness burns is applicable where infection has been eliminated so that daily activity is relatively unaffected. Hydrogels, hydrocolloids, foams and alginates may all have a role to play.

- Hydrogels are comfortable and conformable, provide moisture at the wound bed and can be used with semipermeable films, thus allowing bathing, etc.
- Hydrocolloids are occlusive, need infrequent dressing changes, are comfortable and permit bathing.
- Foams are comfortable and absorbent and some are adhesive.
- Alginates are absorbent and comfortable and can be used with pads or semipermeable films to allow bathing, etc.

Returning to normal activities, such as swimming and sports, may be facilitated by using occlusive dressings. Monitoring of the healing wound may be undertaken by the practice or district nurse in conjunction with the parents, though teenagers may wish to care for their own wounds on a day-to-day basis. Tetanus protection is essential for all types of burns, irrespective of depth. The choice of dressing material will depend on a thorough assessment of the patient, and in particular the lifestyle of the adolescent will need to be taken into consideration.

The long-term consequences of a chemical burn may be disfiguring, with scarring of the affected area. The adolescent and parents may wish to take legal action against the employer if negligence is involved. The Health and Safety Act may be invoked to prevent recurrence of such an accident and procedures for handling chemicals may need to be reviewed.

Nursing model for David

Luckily for David, his employer took the right course of first aid action, although he should have ensured David had adequate Health and Safety advice before he took the job.

Although a partial-thickness burn should heal without scarring, the type of care David receives now may influence the rest of his life. Any injury to a hand, however superficial, should ideally be assessed by a plastic surgeon.

Use Roper's model (Roper et al 1996) to assess David's care (Table 5.2). The assessment reveals that David has the following major problems.

Motor activities

- Cannot wash
- Cannot eat normally
- Cannot work
- Cannot write
- Cannot drive
- Pain.

Table 5.2
Assessment of David's problems (Case study 5.1)

Activities of living	Problem statements
Eliminating	Normal bowel action Urine output Cannot use right hand to attend to personal hygiene following elimination
Eating and drinking	Good diet and fluid intake but cannot eat very well with one hand
Working and playing	Unable to continue work, cannot write as right-handed Future employment/education may be affected
Mobilizing	Just started driving lessons which he cannot continue
Sleeping	Arm and hand still quite painful, cannot get comfortable at night Worried about employment and school work
Personal cleansing	Cannot wash or shower very well
Expressing sexuality	Worried about effects of burns or scarring to his arm and hand

Psychosocial aspects
- Disruption in schooling
- Anxiety
- Self-image (effect of scarring).

PRACTICE POINTS

For an apparently small injury there are many complications.

- The management of the burnt hand can best be achieved with silver sulpha-diazine in a sterile plastic bag; the arm can be covered with a film dressing or other low-adherent material. Neither arm nor hand will require grafting.
- Documentation of treatment and wound assessment must be meticulous in case there are complications at a later date.
- Think about how this accident could have been avoided.

PRESSURE SORES

Pressure ulcers are normally associated with elderly patients but can occur in young patients with disabilities such as spina bifida, as discussed in Case study 5.2.

Case study 5.2

Pressure ulcers in a young, physically disabled teenager

Thirteen-year-old Tracy Childs was born with spina bifida and has been paralysed from the waist down since birth. Incontinent of faeces and urine, Tracy has been hospitalized many times for urinary diversion and now has a permanent urostomy.

Tracy lives with her mother and father and younger brother John, who is seven years old. The family house has been adapted for Tracy's wheelchair and has a downstairs bathroom with shower. Although dogged by episodes of ill health, Tracy remains a cheerful and determined teenager that, with her devoted mother giving 24-hour care, copes well with her disabilities.

Six weeks ago Tracy complained of feeling unwell and was diagnosed as having a urinary infection. Despite a course of oral antibiotics she became nauseated and confused and had a temperature of 40°C. She was rushed into hospital where she received intravenous antibiotics and was, for several days, seriously ill. Unable to eat food, she lost 4.5 kg in weight and because of her position in bed and lack of her usual stoma bags, urine leaked out around her conduit. This resulted on three occasions in Tracy lying in one position for several hours on wet sheets. When she finally became well she was put in an ordinary wheelchair without the pressure-relieving cushion which she would normally have in her wheelchair at home.

Tracy's mother was distressed at the apparent lack of attention to her daughter's needs. Although the staff were caring, the ward was obviously inadequately staffed and lacked what Tracy's mother viewed as essential equipment. On her mother's insistence, Tracy was discharged home as soon as her temperature became normal and prescribed an oral antibiotic regimen. The day after discharge, in the course of a blanket bath, Tracy's mother noticed two broken areas on the teenager's left hip and right ischial tuberosity. Two days later they became black in the middle and deep red around the outside. She was horrified, realizing these were pressure ulcers, and called the general practitioner, who sent the district nurse to assess the situation.

Figure 5.2
Teenager with spina bifida
with a deep undermining
pressure ulcer.

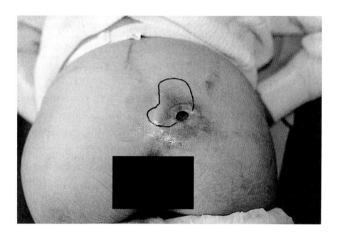

Aetiology

Spina bifida is caused by defective closure of the caudal neuropore towards the end of the fourth week of gestation. Spina bifida occulta (non-fusion of the spinal arches limited to vertebral defects) occurs in around 10% of the population. Although a small dimple or hair tuft can be seen, individuals are generally asymptomatic. However, spina bifida cystica is less common, occurring in 1 in 1000 births. The lesion is sac-like in appearance, with multiple unfused vertebrae. The lesions can be closed, with either the meninges alone (meningocele) or both the meninges and the spinal cord (meningomyelocele) within the sac. A more severe version, myeloschisis, occurs when an open neural tube is present without an overlying sac. Spina bifida causes severe neurological defects corresponding to the level at which the defect is found (National Institute of Neurological Disorders and Stroke 2004).

Children born with high lesions have a poor neurological prognosis and the majority of patients experience both bladder and bowel problems. For children with meningomyelocele, a common complication is hydrocephalus. Owing to their immobility, it is not unusual for these individuals to have many episodes of pressure ulcers (Figure 5.2).

Management

The management of pressure ulcers in children or teenagers with chronic illness or disability needs to address three important issues.

- Maintenance of self-care and independence
- Provision of pressure-relieving and other equipment such as wheelchairs
- Implications of pressure ulcers on the patient's general health and disability.

It needs to be stressed that the effect of having a pressure ulcer will alter the whole lifestyle of the individual. Also the likelihood of further breakdown increases if adequate preventive measures are not put in place as a permanent part of management.

Multiple ulcer development over a period of time will cause further disability, require plastic surgery and predispose to life-threatening systemic infections.

The management of grade IV necrotic pressure ulcers is particularly problematic as the extent of the tissue damage under the necrotic eschar is often hidden. Damage may be superficial or may extend down to muscle and bone.

This is a serious and potentially hazardous situation for a patient where severe and deep-seated infection causes septicaemia and organ failure. Debridement of this devitalized necrotic tissue can be achieved in several ways – surgically, chemically and by autolysis using dressings (see Chapter 8). Tracy may choose a conservative method of treatment that can be carried out at home by the district nurse. A hydrogel used with a semipermeable film in conjunction with sharp debridement of loose devitalized tissue is a common form of treatment.

For chair-bound individuals, a written plan for the use of repositioning devices, negotiated between the individual and the professionals and tailored to the specific needs of the individual, is an effective way of reducing the likelihood of pressure ulcers (Pieper 2000). Included in this type of plan would be consideration of the postural alignment, distribution of weight, balance and stability, and pressure relief.

A seat cushion is essential for providing pressure relief in wheelchairs as very high pressures can be exerted by wheelchair base seats (Dealey 1999). In addition to using an appropriate seat cushion, chair-bound individuals can be taught to relieve pressure by shifting their weight regularly throughout the day. Relief of the high levels of pressure produced by sitting should be undertaken at least hourly. For patients with spinal cord injuries, weight shifts have been shown to be effective in reducing the risk of pressure ulcers (Garber 2004).

The care and management outlined below can be used as a framework for many individuals in similar situations.

Nursing model for Tracy

When assessing and planning Tracy's care, the district nurse must be fully aware of Tracy's previous history. The nurse must also assess the family as a unit and not consider Tracy's needs apart from her family.

Although Tracy has a whole host of medical problems she also is an adolescent who has a right to be considered in all aspects of care (Taylor et al 1999).

Orem's model can assist the nurse in her assessment to instigate the development of family-centred care. The nurse should be seen as the central 'facilitator' of care, not the main caregiver, and should be prepared to let go of tasks that may be seen traditionally as belonging to the nurse.

The first stage of the assessment establishes whether there is a deficit in Tracy's self-care abilities. Remember that we are also assessing Tracy's mother as the main caregiver.

Orem's model uses six universal self-care needs to make the assessment (Table 5.3). Having identified Tracy's problems, the nurse must decide why there is a self-care deficit. Is it due to a lack of knowledge, skills or motivation or a limited range of behaviour? Tracy and her family were living a normal life before this period of hospitalization and they may need to learn new skills or new behaviour in order to resume that normalcy. By recognizing the cause of the problem, the district nurse can plan with Tracy and her mother a new course of action that is suited to all concerned. The amount of intervention the nurse gives at this stage is crucial to the re-establishment of self-caring abilities.

Nursing intervention will be wholly compensatory, partly compensatory or educative/supportive (Table 5.4).

Table 5.3
Assessment of Tracy
(Case study 5.2) using
Orem's model

Self-care need	Self-care ability	Self-care deficit
Sufficient intake of air	Tracy breathes without problems whichever position she is placed in	Nil
Fluid balance	Tracy is required to drink 2–3 litres daily to keep kidneys patent Feels weak following hospitalization	Needs extra fluids (A) Further urinary tract infection (P) Renal failure (P)
Nutrition	Extra energy needed owing to pressure ulcers and weight loss Tracy has never had a large appetite	Weight loss (A) Catabolic state (A) Poor diet (A)
Elimination	Urostomy bag leaking due to weight loss and lying in bed Bowels evacuated daily by manual evacuation	Cannot manage urostomy without leakage (A) Diarrhoea due to antibiotics (P) Increase interface friction (P)
Activity and rest	Has had prolonged period in bed Will continue to spend more time in bed, not in wheelchair owing to pressure ulcers	Inadequate exercise (A) Muscle wasting (P) Non-healing pressure ulcers (A) Further skin breakdown (P)
Socializing	Normally a very sociable girl, Tracy has had a long period in hospital without her usual social contacts Mother has spent long periods in hospital with her	Depressed due to enforced hospitalization (A)
Normalcy	Normally goes to school Family outings Has friends to the house Considers her disability as normal to her	Missed schooling (A) Ill-health stopped family outings (A) Acute illness reinforces her disability (A)
Danger to self	Is able (with her mother's help) to manoeuvre herself in and out of bed and in and out of shower Feels weak and unable to perform normal hygiene or mobility roles	Further breakdown of skin (P) Chest infection (P) Injury to herself and mother (P)

(A), actual problem; (P), potential problem.

Table 5.4
Nursing interventions for Tracy (Case study 5.2)

Self-care deficit	Goal	Interventions
a) Needs extra fluids (lack of skill and motivation) b) Further urinary tract infection c) Renal failure (lack of knowledge)	Tracy can drink as much as she can tolerate with an aim to reach 2 litres daily (PC)	a) Supply of Tracy's favourite drinks to be available at bedside in vacuum flasks or large juice containers. 'Bendy' straws or sealed containers will aid drinking when lying in bed b, c) Discuss level of knowledge of Tracy and her mother regarding the importance of keeping kidneys flushed with fluids. Use simple explanations without frightening them
a) Weight loss (limited range of behaviour) b) Catabolic state c) Poor diet (lack of knowledge)	To regain previous weight (PC) To reduce the effects of catabolism and promote wound healing (PC, ES) To promote a healthier diet for future eating (ES)	a, b) Increase energy content of diet to enhance weight gain, but avoid protein overload of kidneys. Contact community dietician to plan specific diet with family. Discuss with Tracy and her mother effects of catabolism on wound healing c) Plan a diet with the family which will take into account finances, availability of foodstuffs, and likes and dislikes.
a) Cannot manage urostomy bag (limited range of behaviour) b) Diarrhoea due to antibiotic (lack of knowledge) c) Increase of interface friction (lack of knowledge)	Eliminate leakage (WC) Prevent diarrhoea and reduce interface friction (ES)	a) Reassess urostomy bag size and stoma. Refer to stomatherapist for new appliance b) Explain importance of taking antibiotics at correct times. Advise Tracy to report any change in bowel motion c) Reinforce importance of skin cleansing following urine spillage
a) Inadequate exercise (lack of motivation and limited behaviour) b) Muscle wasting (limited behaviour) c) Non-healing pressure ulcers (lack of knowledge) d) Further skin breakdown (lack of knowledge)	To resume 'normal' physical activity level (PC, ES) To heal pressure ulcers (WC) To prevent further ulcer development (ES)	a, b) Resume daily routine of passive exercises of legs while in bed. Sit in chair for increasing periods each day, resuming arm lifts every half-hour. Discuss possibility of community physiotherapy weekly to keep motivation level high c) Reassess Tracy using identified risk assessment tool and review whether pressure-relieving equipment (bed and chair) meets her needs Document wound position, size and tissue characteristics. Trace and/or photograph. Debride wound, using dressing material that will (i) keep wound occluded and prevent infection, (ii) minimize dressing changes, (iii) be possible for the mother to change if necessary, and (iv) provide comfort for the patient d) Discuss with Tracy and her mother the reasons for initial ulcer development and indicators for prevention of future breakdown
a) Depressed owing to enforced hospitalization (lack of knowledge)	To introduce positive outlook on life (ES)	a) Encourage Tracy and her mother to reflect on the reasons why she went into hospital. Highlight the benefits of being home. Allow Tracy to work through her feelings, giving her time to talk

PRACTICE POINTS

- In this case the district nurse's role has been mainly educative and partially compensatory. Even the wound care can be increasingly transferred to the mother.
- However, care must be taken that this role is willingly taken on. Often an acute episode like this triggers a breakdown in the family as the care unit.
- The nurse must assess the environment carefully and look for indications of strain and stress.

ROAD TRAFFIC ACCIDENTS

Road traffic accidents are a common cause of traumatic wounds in teenagers and the associated problems are illustrated in Case study 5.3.

Case study 5.3

Road traffic accident

Darren Adams had been employed as a motorbike courier for the last six months. Although he left school with three A-levels, he was unable to find employment for 12 months. Despite the job being unsuited to his capabilities, he was pleased to have some form of income until the right job came along.

Darren has always liked drinking with his friends but has usually been sensible enough to walk or take a taxi home. Last Friday, however, it was raining heavily and he did not have any money left for a taxi so he decided to ride his bike home. The roads were slippery and at a junction Darren pulled out in front of a car. The car braked but skidded into the bike, knocking Darren into the air some two metres before he landed on the bonnet of the car.

Darren was rushed to the local accident and emergency department. He was conscious, having sustained a fractured femur and severe lacerations to face and arm. Following admission, Darren was informed that the police wished to interview him, at which point he became abusive and tried to throw himself off the trolley.

Epidemiology

In the UK in 2001, 34.5 people per billion passenger kilometres were killed on bicycles and motorcycles accounted for a further 122.7 people killed per billion kilometres (Department of Transport 2004). Others experienced serious injuries. Head injuries are more common in young males than females in a ratio of 3:1, mostly affecting the 16–35 age group. In the UK 5000 young people per annum will be expected to die of their head injuries, though many of these injuries are preventable. The use of crash helmets for motorcyclists and safety belts in cars has resulted in less serious injuries. A common factor that contributes to head injuries is overconsumption of alcohol (Allan 1999).

Management

Many patients seen in accident and emergency departments are fit, young individuals. Irrespective of the wound size, accurate assessment, diagnosis and thorough wound toilet must be achieved to ensure that any deficit in wound healing is identified and the appropriate treatment given.

Before assessment of the traumatic wound is made, the patient's condition must be stabilized. Standard assessments of airway, breathing and circulation are made to ensure that all life threatening conditions are identified. Any external bleeding is controlled with direct pressure on the wound. A thorough history of how the accident happened is then recorded, though this is difficult where a patient is unconsciousness and there are no witnesses. Other factors that are taken into account are:

- exact mechanism of injury
- amount of force
- foreign bodies in wound
- tendon or nerve damage
- time and place of accident.

It is important to establish whether the patient has any medical history of diabetes mellitus or epilepsy, is allergic to or is taking any particular medication.

Wound assessment and cleansing

All traumatic wounds will be contaminated by the time the patient arrives in the accident and emergency department (Bale & Leaper 2000) so an aseptic technique is not necessary until removal of gross contaminants is achieved (Dealey 1999). The following is recommended practice:

- Foreign material should be removed by washing (irrigation) (see Chapter 3), brushing or with forceps.
- Before further investigation is attempted the wound must be anaesthetized with plain lignocaine.
- Remove all deeply embedded foreign bodies and examine the damage in relation to underlying nerves and tendons (Bale & Leaper 2000).
- Debridement of traumatized and devitalized tissue must be carried out, remembering that wound toilet should be directly proportional to the extent of contamination (Ayello et al 2004).

Investigation

Radiographic investigations of traumatized limbs and suspected injury sites are required for an accurate diagnosis.

Antibiotics

Antibiotics are indicated for:

- badly contaminated wounds
- human or animal bites
- diabetic or immunocompromised patients.

Tetanus prophylaxis

Tetanus prophylaxis may be considered for wounds more than six hours old that display:

- large amounts of devitalized tissue
- deep puncture-type injury such as a stab wound

Table 5.5
Assessment of Darren's problems (Case study 5.3) using Roy's adaptation model

Life area	Assessment Level 1 – Behaviour	Assessment Level 2 – Stimuli		
		Focal	Contextual	Residual
Self-concept	Abusive violent behaviour Fear of surroundings	Confrontation with A&E staff Still in shock	Staff not experienced in handling patient A&E department	Social stigma of drunk driver Never previously hospitalized
Role/function	Fears loss of job Fears police conviction	Major traumatic injury Knows he should not have driven	Extent of injury not assessed	No previous involvement with law
Interdependency	Dependent on staff, lack of self-control	Helpless owing to injuries and alcohol	Sudden change from being well to being seriously ill	Not 'normal' level of behaviour
Regulation	Multiple lacerations to face and arms Pain Contamination from road	Contaminated wounds Compound fracture of femur Infection in wound	Wounds embedded with grit and dirt from road Further damage to underlying tissue Length of time before arrival in A&E	
Oxygenation	Hyperventilation	Fear and shock	Pain in leg	
Nutrition	Feeling nauseated	Pain in leg Shock	Effects of alcohol	

- contact with soil or manure (e.g. in farm workers)
- evidence of infection
- human or animal bites (Bale & Leaper 2000).

Nursing model for Darren

Darren has sustained major injuries and requires a great deal of immediate treatment. Unfortunately for him, his arrival in the accident and emergency department has commenced with a confrontational event that is not conducive to developing a relationship with the nursing staff.

The nurse needs to calm Darren before treatment can begin and an assessment of his needs undertaken. The nurse should also consider the psychological consequences of labelling Darren as a drunken driver.

Darren has experienced a sudden change in circumstances from being a fit, healthy, intelligent young man. He is now immobile, facing criminal charges and labelled as being 'stupid' with no regard for other lives. In other words, he will need to adapt to ill health. Roy's adaptation model (Roy & Andrews 1999) may be used to assess and outline a plan of care (Table 5.5).

PRACTICE POINTS

- Before Darren can have an assessment of his traumatic injuries, the staff need to calm him as he is in grave danger of adding to his injuries.
- Look at the assessment of his psychosocial status and identify the major problems:
  violent behaviour due to *shock, fear* and effects of *alcohol*
  placed in hospital surroundings which are *new* to him
  does not have any *family or friends* to provide *support.*

How can these problems be resolved?

Because of the way in which the traumatic injuries are incurred, patients are suddenly plunged into what may seem a hostile environment in the accident and emergency unit. This is compounded in Darren's case as the police are also there waiting to see him.

Darren's wounds were debrided, irrigated and sutured. Antibiotic cover and frequent wound observation were instituted for the prevention and early detection of wound infection. In the long term the extent of Darren's scarring could have a lasting effect on his psychological state. Facial wounds often require the skills of a plastic surgeon using careful suturing techniques (see Chapter 4).

Most accident and emergency departments operate a triage system, enabling staff to prioritize patient care. Those requiring immediate emergency treatment are attended to first, while less urgent cases are dealt with later. In this case it might have been advisable to assess Darren's injuries and gain his confidence before the police were mentioned.

The priority of management is to ensure there are no life-threatening problems by using the 'ABC' protocol (airway, breathing and circulation), checking that there are no major bleeding points at the site of fracture and assessing previous blood loss. Monitor vital signs for signs of shock. Calm the patient with:

- reassurance: talk slowly, in a quiet area away from the hustle and bustle of the department. Enlist his trust – the nurse is there to help him
- pain relief: give appropriate analgesia, if vital signs are satisfactory. Local analgesia may also be required before wound toilet is commenced at site of fracture
- explanation: explain the necessity to assess his injuries as quickly as possible and that this will require his cooperation. Ask him if he would like his family contacted.

Accident and emergency department staff are trained to provide reassurance and gain the patient's trust quickly, while simultaneously performing resuscitation techniques.

Look at the physiological areas of assessment. The important points here are:

- wound cleansing and wound toilet
- thorough examination of lacerations and extent of injuries
- antibiotic and tetanus cover
- accurate documentation of both events of accident and nature of injury.

Devise the care plan, taking these points into account. Look at the assessment in Table 5.5 if you need help.

SUMMARY

Injury to teenagers can be traumatic both physiologically and psychologically. The nurse has an important role to play in providing skilled management of the wound and gaining the patient's trust. The bond that can develop between nurse and teenager can be rewarding and enhance the level of care given.

The important issues to remember when dealing with the cases outlined can be summarized as follows.

- Gain the trust of the teenager before commencement of any treatment.
- Ensure that adequate pain relief is always given.
- Consider the effects that immobility or scarring may have on them for the rest of their lives.
- Be aware that teenagers can easily be emotionally crushed; always communicate in a clear and understanding way.
- Documentation, as always, is of utmost importance. Claims may be made many years on from the actual date of the accident or injury.
- Be aware that inadequate management may result in inadequate wound healing.

FURTHER READING

Gowar J P, Lawrence J C 1995 The incidence, cause and treatment of minor burns. Journal of Wound Care 4(2): 71–74.

Wardrope J, Smith J 1993 The management of wounds and burns. Oxford University Press, Oxford.

Wright B 1993 Caring in crisis: a handbook of intervention skills, 2nd edn. Churchill Livingstone, Edinburgh.

REFERENCES

Allan D 1999 The nervous system. In: Alexander M R, Fawcett J N, Runciman P J (eds) Nursing practice. Churchill Livingstone, Edinburgh.

Ayello E A, Baranoski S, Kerstein M D, Cuddigan J 2004 Wound debridement. In: Baranoski S, Ayello E A (eds) Wound care essentials: practice principles. Lippincott, Williams and Wilkins, Springhouse, Pennsylvania.

Bale S, Leaper D 2000 Acute wounds. In: Bale S, Harding K, Leaper D (eds) An introduction to wounds. Emap Healthcare Ltd, London.

Childstats 2004 America's children 2002: adolescent mortality rates. Available online at: www.childstats.gov. Accessed 28.08.04.

Dealey C 1999 The management of patients with chronic wounds. In: The care of wounds. Blackwell Science, Oxford.

Department of Transport 2004 Passenger death rates by mode of transport. Available online at: www.statistics.gov.uk. Accessed 24.08.04.

Dowsett C 2002 The assessment and management of burns. British Journal of Community Nursing 7(5): 230–239.

Garber S L 2004 Spinal cord injury population. In: Baranoski S, Ayello E A (eds) Wound care essentials: practice principles. Lippincott, Williams and Wilkins, Springhouse, Pennsylvania.

Hazinski M F 1999 Manual of pediatric critical care. Mosby, St Louis, Missouri.

Health and Safety Executive 2004 Injuries to workers. Available online at: www.statistics.gov.uk. Accessed 24.08.04.

Lawrence J C 1990 Burn and scald injuries. Topic Briefing HS40. RoSPA, Birmingham.

McCormack A, La Hei E R, Martin H C 2003 First-aid management of minor burns in children: a prospective study of children presenting to the Children's Hospital at Westmead, Sydney. Medical Journal of Australia 178(1): 31–33.

Mertens D M, Jenkins M E, Warden G D 1997 Outpatient burns management. Nursing Clinics of North America 32 (2): 343–364.

National Institute of Neurological Disorders and Stroke 2004 NINDS spina bifida information page. Available online at: www.sbaa.org. Accessed 28.08.04.

Page R M 2002 Towards social inclusion. In: Ward H, Rose W (eds) Approaches to needs assessment in children's services. Jessica Kingsley Publishers, London.

Petch N, Cason C G 1993 Examining first aid received by burn and scald patients. Journal of Wound Care 2(2): 102–105.

Pieper B 2000 Mechanical forces: pressure, shear, and friction. In: Bryant R A (ed) Acute and chronic wounds: nursing management. Mosby, St Louis, Missouri.

Roper N, Logan W W, Tierney A J 1996 The elements of nursing, 4th edn. Churchill Livingstone, Edinburgh.

Roy C, Andrews H 1999 The Roy adaptation model, 2nd edn. Appleton and Lange, Stamford, Connecticut.

Taylor J, Muller D, Wattley L, Harris P 1999 The adolescent in hospital. In: Nursing children. Stanley Thornes, London.

Wheal A 1999 Adolescents. In: Adolescence: positive approaches for working with young people. Russell House Publishing, Lyme Regis, Dorset.

6

Wound care in the young adult

KEY ISSUES   This chapter examines the type of wound management required by the young adult.

Clinical Case Studies
Aetiology and management of:

■ A 22-year-old man requiring emergency excision of a pilonidal sinus
■ A woman requiring an emergency caesarean section who encounters wound problems postoperatively
■ A 36-year-old man with a traumatic injury following an accident that requires preparation for plastic surgery
■ A 34-year-old mother with osteosarcoma of the leg
■ A self-inflicted leg wound.

Nursing Models
Examples of their application to practice are taken from:

■ Orem's model
■ Roy's adaptation model
■ Riehl-Sisca's interaction model

PRACTICE POINTS   As you read through this chapter concentrate on the following:

■ the effects emergency surgery may have on postoperative wound management
■ factors that should be considered in preoperative management that enhance postoperative care
■ the effect a wound can have on the patient's normal living pattern
■ the range of dressings available that patients can manage themselves
■ the importance of including the patient in planning care.

INTRODUCTION   Young adulthood is a stage in the life-cycle where the individual feels immune to disease and ill health. The young value their youthfulness and vigour and generally thrive on fitness. For the young, the image of a sick individual may be one of a helpless, older person being the passive recipient of both medical and nursing care. This age group would challenge this image and feel confident, empowered and expect to become involved in making decisions about their care and management. Patients and health professionals are encouraged to work together in partnership (Coulter 2000, McQueen 2000), so that patients have the opportunity to make informed choices about their care. Nurses should ensure that, as with all patients, young adults are engaged in making decisions about their wound care.

PREPARING FOR PLANNED SURGERY

Surgical procedures may be offered to many young people with a variety of health problems. For many problems that are not life threatening the decision to accept or refuse surgery rests solely with the individual. Examples of these problems include lipomas and ingrowing toenails; the patient will decide how troublesome it is. Other health problems such as inguinal hernia, ovarian cyst and pilonidal sinus may lead to further complications and are best treated with surgical intervention. Individuals vary greatly in their response to the prospect of surgery: some regard it in a matter-of-fact way, others with great fear and trepidation. Experiences in childhood or the experiences of family members or friends can be an influencing factor.

Great advances have been made in surgical procedures. The use of the laparoscope for 'keyhole' surgery has enabled knee surgery and abdominal surgery to be carried out through very small incisions. Where appropriate, such operations can take place in day surgery units where the patient need not stay overnight. From a cost-saving point of view, there is an increasing trend for young, fit individuals to be offered day surgery. From the patient's point of view, the advantages include a short stay in hospital, reduced pain and immobility, and an earlier return to normal activities.

Patients requiring more extensive surgery will need to be admitted to a surgical ward. Preoperatively the nurse has an important role to play in helping to prepare the patient for surgery. As well as the physical assessment, the nurse can provide information and emotional support on admission. It is well documented that with information and support given to reduce stress and anxiety, the patient has a much better postoperative outcome (Rodgers 1999).

With planning, education need not be disrupted and it is usual for young patients to be offered a date for surgery to coincide with university and college holidays. Interruption of daily activities may be perceived as problematic for the young individual. Concern may be focused around the length of time that a favourite sport may not be played or when they may be able to socialize. Linked to this may be concerns about an altered body image. The young value their youth, health, beauty and vigour (Smitherman 1981) and any disfigurement, however minor, may have a negative effect.

COPING WITH EMERGENCY SURGERY

The onset of an acute illness or trauma can result in the need for emergency surgery. An example is given in Case study 6.1. Preparation of the young person as described above may not be possible and often only brief, essential information can be given in the immediate preoperative period. In the postoperative period patients are likely to have many questions, which could need answering several times as the patient recovers from both the anaesthesia and surgery.

Case study 6.1

Emergency excision of pilonidal sinus

Colin Sharples is a 22-year-old law student just entering his final year of studies. A fit, healthy young man who has always been involved in many sporting activities, he has never had any experience of illness or hospitalization.

During the past six months he has had a feeling of discomfort in his natal cleft which appears to come and go and is often associated with feeling generally unwell. Last week the discomfort became an acute, stabbing pain which prevented him from sitting down. He went to the college doctor who diagnosed his condition as pilonidal disease and gave him a course of antibiotics. Colin unfortunately took his antibiotics for two days only as he felt better and did not really like taking tablets. Within a week he was admitted to hospital for an emergency wide excision of a pilonidal abscess.

Following surgery the wound was left to heal by secondary intention and measured 10 cm in length by 3 cm breadth and 4 cm depth. Colin was extremely anxious postoperatively and, although in pain, was reluctant to stay in hospital as he wanted to resume his studies.

Aetiology

Pilonidal sinus disease commonly affects young adults, arising at some time after puberty, and is rarely found after the age of 40 years. Men are affected by pilonidal sinus disease around ten times more than women and it is associated with having a sedentary occupation, a family history, obesity and local irritation or trauma prior to onset of symptoms (Miller & Harding 2003). Around 75% of those undergoing surgery are males and 25% are females (Bascom 1994). Pilonidal sinus disease causes a great deal of suffering, inconvenience, loss of time from work and loss of income, as patients can have problems for up to three years. Patients generally present with recurrent pain and purulent discharge (Senapati & Cripps 2000). The recurrence rate following excision can be as high as 50% (Jones 1992) and with reconstructive skin flaps as low as 5% (Kitchen 1996).

There are several theories as to why pilonidal sinus disease occurs, the most likely being acquired disease (Figure 6.1). With the onset of puberty, sex hormones begin to act on pilosebaceous glands in the natal cleft. With this a hair follicle becomes distended with **keratin** and subsequently infected, so resulting in a folliculitis and an abscess that extends down into subcutaneous fat (Miller & Harding 2003). In 93% the direction of the abscess and secondary tracts follows the orientation of the inflamed hair follicles. The abscess is likely to drain out onto the skin through the tract (Berry 1992). Hairs are drilled or sucked into the abscess cavity through friction with movement of the buttocks. This process encourages loose debris and other body hair to enter and accumulate in the sinus (Figure 6.2). Most commonly *Staphylococcus aureus* and *Bacteroides* are the pathogens causing the infection. Patients may be asymptomatic for some time before presenting with local discomfort and/or discharge. However, about 50% of patients present with an acute pilonidal abscess.

Figure 6.1
(a) Pilonidal sinus; (b) pilonidal abscess; (c) a combination of pilonidal sinus with pilonidal abscess.

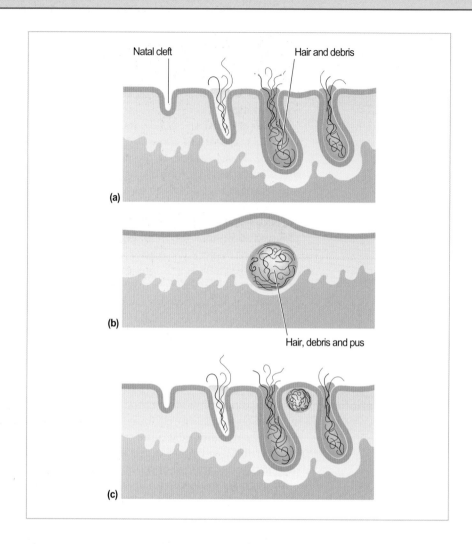

Management

There are a number of surgical techniques available, although no one procedure has been demonstrated to be better than another overall. It is generally agreed that the most effective emergency management of a pilonidal abscess is simple incision and drainage (Miller & Harding 2003). However, the treatment of chronic and recurrent pilonidal disease is more difficult and the options include excision with primary closure or healing by secondary intention, Lord's procedure, phenol injections and skin flaps (Duxbury et al 2003, Khairi & Brown 1995 Senapati et al 2000).

Several treatments may be offered to patients.

- Curettage for small, non-infected sinuses: it may be possible to remove the hairs with a pair of forceps and brushing out tracts. Lord's procedure is one such treatment that is reported to be associated with 80–90% healing (Senapati & Cripps 2000).

Figure 6.2
Pilonidal sinus disease prior to surgery. Marked on the patient's skin is the area to be excised, together with the sites of individual sinuses.

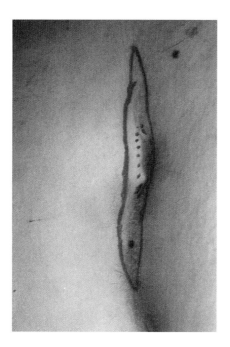

- Excision and primary closure: here the sinuses are excised and the wound edges brought together and sutured. These procedures can result in 70% healing at two weeks, although some 20% develop a wound infection (Khairi & Brown 1995, Kitchen 1996, Peterson et al 2002, Senapati et al 2000).
- Wide excision and laying open of the sinuses together with the skin: all tissues are excised down to the sacrum (Miller & Harding 2003). The patient requires frequent dressing changes and a great deal of support. This procedure is associated with 70–90% healing at 70 days and 5–15% recurrence rates (Senapati & Cripps 2000).

As Colin's disease was widespread the wide excision technique was used, leaving a large cavity wound (Figures 6.3–6.6).

Local wound management
This large cavity will take about 6–8 weeks to heal by secondary intention. With a little care Colin could return to fairly normal activities quickly and could take responsibility for his own wound hygiene. Some of the dressing materials that could be used include the following.

- Day 0–2: alginate materials, especially those containing sodium, are useful haemostatic agents. The dressing can be packed into the wound immediately following surgery, in the operating theatre, to achieve haemostasis. After 48 hours this alginate packing can be washed out of the cavity using warm saline.
- Day 2 through the proliferative phase: alginate and hydrofibre materials can be used but this treatment needs a nurse to change the dressings. Other useful materials include cavity foam dressings and occasionally a hydrogel. Foam dressings, especially disposable and those formed in situ, can be

Figure 6.3
Wide excision of pilonidal
sinus at week 2.

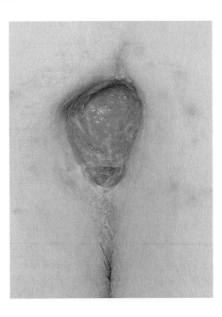

Figure 6.4
At week 4.

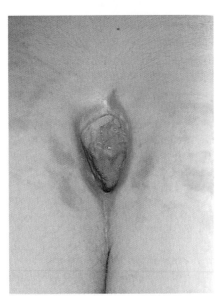

managed by patients on a daily basis and so facilitate early return to normal activity. The main function of a cavity dressing for a pilonidal sinus excision is to keep the wound edges apart as healing takes place, so preventing superficial bridges and the possibility of a dead space in the depths of the wound. Wound hygiene is of particular importance as is regular inspection and assessment of the granulation tissue to detect the early signs of clinical infection (Miller & Harding 2003). Here, the signs of clinical infection include the presence of flimsy, friable, discoloured granulation tissue, bleeding, superficial bridging, pain and increased exudate production (Cutting & White 2004).

Figure 6.5
At week 6.

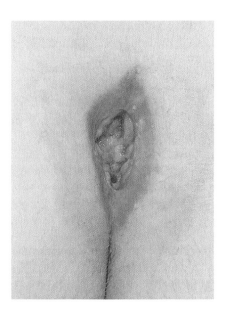

Figure 6.6
At week 8 – healed.

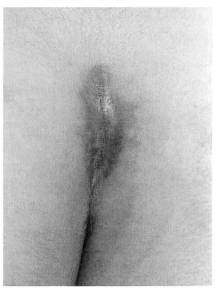

Nursing model for Colin

Colin is a normal, fit, healthy young adult who does not really want to be in hospital or have his normal routine altered. What do you see as his main concerns?

- Disruption of his studies
- Disruption of his sporting activities
- Disruption of sexual activity
- Embarrassment at exposing buttocks to nurses
- Lack of privacy in hospital
- Likelihood of recurrence of disease
- Time of discharge from hospital.

Colin's major worries are not directly concerned with wound management. In a fit, healthy young man this open granulating wound should heal easily and without complication.

PRACTICE POINTS

You should have identified Colin's self-care deficit from the list of main concerns. The management that Colin needs, therefore, should follow these lines.

- Following an initial 3–4 days in hospital Colin can be discharged with arrangements made with the community nurse or university campus nurse to continue care.
- Initially the wound could be packed with alginates to achieve haemostasis; then, in the next few days, a cavity foam dressing could be introduced. Colin could change these dressings himself, following daily showering. He needs to understand that strenuous exercise must be avoided for up to 12 weeks.
- Colin requires a flexible approach to his care, the need to feel in control and the assurance that he has professional advice when needed.
- Orem's model would fulfil these needs, with an early discharge into the community under the care of the university campus nurse and specialist outpatient visits at frequent intervals.

CAESAREAN SECTION

Case study 6.2 discusses the problems arising from wound breakdown after an apparently straightforward caesarean section.

Case study 6.2

Caesarean section

Mrs Kate Hemmings, a 34-year-old, gave birth to her third child by emergency caesarean section. Kate had a caesarean delivery with her first child but delivered her second child normally and had wanted to try and deliver this baby normally also. Following seven days in hospital, Kate and baby Julia were discharged home into the care of the community staff.

Her sutures were removed at 10 days with the wound apparently having healed without any complications. She felt well in herself, albeit a little tired, but felt this was to be expected with a small baby and two other toddlers to cope with.

By the 12th day she noticed a small red spot in the middle of the scar line which, following a bath, began to ooze fluid. Alarmed at this, she called the district nurse who placed a dressing pad on the area.

Over the next week the oozing continued and an opening became visible which measured 2 cm in width when probed. The surrounding wound area was hard and red and Kate was feeling generally unwell. The district nurse probed the wound and found it undermined 1 cm either side of the scar line (Figure 6.7). The nurse called the general practitioner who admitted Kate to the gynaecology ward at the local hospital. The wound was opened up 1.5 cm either side of the gaping edge to make a small cavity to facilitate drainage of exudate (Figures 6.8–6.10). The wound was packed with an alginate dressing and on Kate's insistence, she was discharged home 48 hours later.

Figure 6.7
Kate Hemmings' wound, showing a probe inserted into the undermining area.

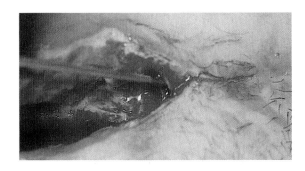

Figure 6.8
Local anaesthetic being injected into the area to be incised.

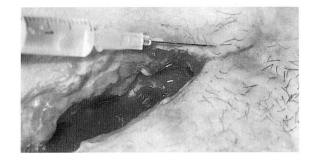

Figure 6.9
Incising the undermined area.

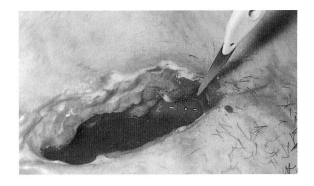

Figure 6.10
The resultant cavity wound is now a suitable shape for healing by secondary intention.

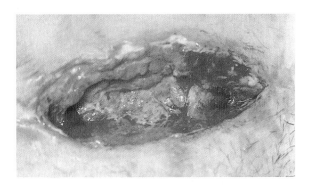

Figure 6.11
The lower uterine segment has been excised transversely and the large fetal head, directly occipitoposterior, has been delivered by manual extraction (reproduced with kind permission from Beischer & Mackay 1986).

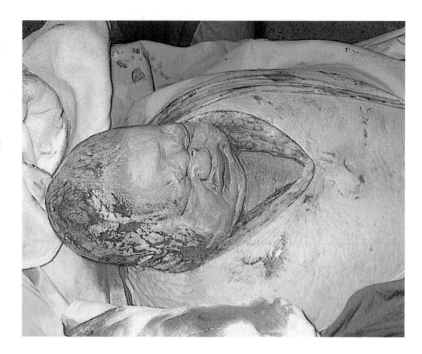

Aetiology

Normal spontaneous vaginal delivery remains constant at around 66% of all births in the UK (Thomas & Paranjothy 2001). Caesarean section is the operation by which a potentially viable fetus is delivered through an incision in the abdominal wall and uterus. It is indicated for fetal compromise, failure to progress in labour (dystocia), previous caesarean section and breech presentation (Thomas & Paranjothy 2001). However, a matter of concern is the gradual increase in the incidence of caesarean section in the UK to around 21.5% of deliveries, and national guidelines have been developed to help ensure that only those women who need the procedure on good clinical grounds receive it (NICE 2004a). The guidelines recommend that when indicated, the benefits, risks and the evidence base for different interventions of caesarean section should be discussed with the woman and also where women request a caesarean section without good clinical reason. In order to decrease morbidity from caesarean section, regional anaesthesia should be used in conjunction with antibiotic prophylaxis, antacids and antiemetics (NICE 2004a).

The most common surgical technique employed is the lower segment caesarean section (Figure 6.11). A transverse abdominal incision 3 cm above the symphysis pubis is the technique of choice as this is associated with shorter operating times, reduced bleeding, reduced postoperative morbidity and pain, and an improved cosmetic effect (NICE 2004a). Postoperative infection is also reduced because the lower segment is outside the peritoneal cavity.

Management

Normally wound management would entail removal of sutures at between 10 and 14 days. Here, however, as with breakdown of surgical wounds, it is advisable to incise the wound to allow free drainage of exudate (see Chapter 3).

This type of wound can be managed using an alginate packing dressing, gently inserted into the undermining wound. The function of the dressing in

Table 6.1
Assessment of Mrs
Hemmings' problems
(Case study 6.2) using
Orem's model

Self-care need	Self-care ability	Self-care deficit
Nutrition	Little time to eat with three children	Inadequate diet (A)
	Little appetite owing to infection	Anaemia (P)
	Losing nutrients through breast-feeding	Unable to breast-feed (P)
Activity and rest	Not sleeping because of new baby	Delay in wound healing due to lack of sleep (A)
	Worried infection will be passed to baby	Unable to play with children and baby
Socializing	Unable to go out with baby owing to wound infection	Depression (P)
		No normal mother–baby activities (A)
Normalcy	Needs to wait in for nurse to do dressings	Feels restricted
		Cannot get into routine with other children and baby

(A), actual problem; (P), potential problem.

this situation is to maintain a channel through which infected exudate can drain and to allow the wound to heal from its depths. It is probably advisable to irrigate the cavity daily with water or saline, prior to repacking. This will rinse out any fragments of alginate left in the wound and also flush away bacteria. Alternatively, a hydrogel could be introduced into the wound to act as packing. Again, daily irrigation would be beneficial.

Nursing model for Kate

It is obvious that Kate has a postoperative wound infection that requires immediate treatment. However, having had to leave her baby, two young children and husband at home, she insisted on returning home within 48 hours.

It is important to provide her with a flexible form of management that allows her to cope at home. She needs to feel in control of her own care but obviously requires support both emotionally and physically from family and health professions.

Before choosing a model of care, ask yourself the following questions.

- Will Kate be able, or want, to do the dressing herself?
- How will the presence of the wound infection affect the young baby?
- What were the possible reasons for her developing this infection?
- Why is it better that Kate stays at home during her recovery?

Orem's model (Orem 1995) would address Kate's problems, as she will probably be motivated to achieve self-care (Table 6.1).

PRACTICE POINT   You must plan the management in such a way that Kate can resume her way of life as quickly as possible.

TRAUMATIC INJURY

The nature of traumatic injury results in a shocked and seriously ill patient who needs emergency surgery followed by preparation for planned plastic surgery, as in the example in Case study 6.3.

Case study 6.3

Emergency and planned surgery

Mr Jeremy Watkins is a married man of 36 years of age with three children aged 10, 7 and 3. Most of his adult life he has enjoyed water sports although since the children arrived, he is now free to pursue this interest only a few times a year.

He was with two friends taking a 3-day water sports holiday in Wales and canoeing down a river when his canoe overturned and he was crushed against sharp rocks. His friends and the instructor rushed to his assistance to find him shocked, bleeding heavily from his right thigh and on the verge of unconsciousness. The instructor and his friends dragged him out of the water and off the rocks, applied pressure to the large gash and summoned help. On admission to hospital, Jeremy was found to have lost some muscle and subcutaneous fat and skin from his thigh as well as a significant amount of blood. He was transfused and taken to theatre where an orthopaedic surgeon and a plastic surgeon assessed the damage to his leg. Due to the extensive tissue damage, primary closure was not possible and the damaged muscle, fat and skin was debrided, the wound irrigated and a haemostatic alginate packing applied. The wound measured 15 cm long by 16 cm wide and 13 cm deep with no bone involvement and no fractures. By the time Jeremy returned from the recovery room, his wife had travelled 60 miles to be with him, leaving their children with friends.

Aetiology

In the age group 26–45 for the year 2001, around 10% of all water sports injuries, some 610 out of a total of 6000 accidents, were reported to be related to rowing, boating and sailing (American Canoe Association 2004). The same report found that all sports were associated with 116 fatalities, of which 19% were related to water sports. The American Canoe Association (2004) reported that approximately 83% of all canoeing-related fatality victims were not wearing a life jacket at the time of the accident and that occupant movement and weight shift within a canoe played a major role in roughly 50% of all canoeing accidents.

Management

Following surgical excision of the detvitalized skin, muscle and subcutaneous tissues, the wound is packed for 48–72 hours to achieve haemostasis; haemostatic alginate dressings are useful for this purpose. As the wound is extensive, copious amounts of wound exudate are produced. A comfortable, soft, absorbent dressing that can be used throughout most of the healing phase is a hydrophilic foam which is packed into the wound. Without the loss of muscle and subcutaneous tissue, Jeremy would have been able to achieve complete healing using dressings and could have been discharged from hospital a few days postoperatively. However, due to the extensive loss of tissue, Jeremy was referred to the plastic surgeon for reconstructive plastic surgery. The plastic surgeon needed to perform a myocutaneous rotation flap, replacing the defect with muscle and tissue from adjacent areas. In order to control the excessive exudate, prepare the wound bed and ensure that no infection would jeopardize this surgery, it was decided to use topical negative pressure. The VAC system was obtained under the trust's equipment provision contract and applied to the wound for 12 days. Following this treatment the wound bed was clean, healthy and granulating and Jeremy was transferred to his local hospital which had a plastic surgery unit attached to it.

In the immediate postoperative period movement is likely to be difficult and painful but as time passes this will dramatically improve. Provision of adequate, regular analgesia and gentle repositioning will help keep Jeremy as comfortable as possible.

Nursing model for Jeremy

Look back at Jeremy's case. What are the important features that stand out about this patient?

- He has endured *shock* and distress due to the unexpected nature of his accident.
- He has *dependent children.*
- He has undergone emergency surgery and has *waited* almost two weeks for this operation.
- He *needs/wants* to go *home.*
- He has *limited* range of *movement.*

Jeremy needs to go home but will require much support from the community nurses. He is a strong, determined man, used to be completely independent, therefore problems could develop if he chooses not to follow the community nurse's advice on wound care.

- The nurse learns the nature of the difficulty the patient is experiencing.
- The nurse and patient develop a mutual trust.
- The nurse can then identify the patient's problems.

PRACTICE POINT   Using the SOAP assessment framework (Chapter 2), plan Jeremy's care.

Figure 6.12
Fungating osteosarcoma
of the tibia.

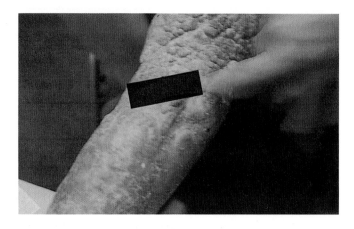

**MALIGNANT
TUMOURS**

*The problems of terminal disease are discussed in relation to an unsuccessfully treated
osteosarcoma (Case study 6.4).*

Case study 6.4

Osteosarcoma of the tibia

Fiona Starr, a 34-year-old mother of two small children, has
osteosarcoma of the tibia and is in the terminal stages of the disease.

Following diagnosis three years ago, Fiona decided on a course of
chemotherapy and radiotherapy rather than a below-knee amputation. Initially
the treatment appeared successful and the tumour shrank in size.
Unfortunately, six months ago the tumour reappeared with a vengeance and,
despite a further course of chemotherapy, began to **fungate** and ulcerate.

The whole of the lower leg is now affected with a fungating mass, is
swollen due to lymphoedema and is painful to touch (Figure 6.12). The
malignancy has infiltrated to the lymphatic system and there is involvement of
the organs of the pelvic region.

Fiona has chosen to be nursed in a hospice setting where her family have
free access. She is fully aware of her prognosis but has difficulty coming to
terms with her initial decision of refusing surgery, as this would probably have
halted the disease process.

Aetiology

Malignant tumours are made up of cells which are able to invade adjacent
tissues but are also able to leave the original site and disseminate to other areas
and form metastases. There are three major groups of cancers:

- Carcinomas: arise in endodermal or ectodermal tissue
- Sarcomas: mesodermal in origin
- Leukaemias/lymphomas: derived from white blood cells and the monocyte-
  macrophage system.

Osteosarcoma is the most common primary malignancy of bone, accounting
for around 56% of all bony tumours (Gurney et al 1995). It is highly aggressive and usually occurs in teenagers and young adults between the ages of 15
and 25 years (Miller et al 1996). Osteosarcoma most commonly occurs in the

lower end of the femur, the upper end of the tibia or the upper end of the humerus (Kramarova & Stiller 1996). These tumours arise in young people and present as swelling of the affected area with or without vague aching. A plain X-ray film shows an increase in radiolucency associated with bone expansion, triangular areas of new bone formation at the periosteal margin and a 'sunray' appearance due to new bone being formed (Link & Eiler 1997). Metastases are rapidly borne by blood to the lung and the survival rate at five years is likely to be less than 10%.

As the disease progresses the cancer may spread into the lymphatic system and also ulcerate through the skin to form a fungating mass. Malodour, increased exudate production, bleeding or fear of bleeding and asymmetry are common problems caused by the fungating mass.

Management

The young person may feel socially isolated and experience altered body image and sexual difficulties as a result. The skilful use of dressing materials can cope with the physical problems of odour, bleeding and excess exudate. Bleeding can be controlled with haemostatic alginate dressings and odour can be controlled with topical use of metronidazole gel that quickly and effectively acts against anaerobic organisms. It can be applied daily at dressing changes until the odour is no longer noticeable. Charcoal dressings absorb odour but need to be held in close contact with the wound or primary dressing to be effective.

At a palliative level these physical symptoms can be managed. The psychological issues are far more difficult to deal with. Impending death is not an easy issue for the young and the interaction between the patient, the family and the professional team is of vital importance.

Nursing model for Fiona

The demands placed on Fiona and on those who care for her during her illness require special assessment from the nurse in order to provide the right type of care. Roy's adaptation model (Roy & Andrews 1999) is designed to help the nurse identify the patient's problems and promote the patient's ability to adapt and cope with them.

Look at one of Fiona's adaptation systems as identified by Roy – the *self-concept system*. This is the view the individual holds of herself both physically and psychologically. What problems of adaptation do you think she has?

Table 6.2 lists some of the stressors causing problems. Look next at the level 2 assessment in Table 6.3 which are caused by focal, contextual or residual stimuli.

Table 6.2
Assessment of Fiona Starr's self-concept system (Case study 6.4)

Life area	Assessment Level 1 – Behaviour
Self-concept	
a) Physical	i) Cannot look at the swollen, fungating, malodorous leg
	ii) Cannot get away from wound – constantly living (dying) with it
b) Psychological	i) Feelings of guilt, e.g. depriving family of mother and wife, should have chosen other treatment option
	ii) Loss of body image and feelings of mutilation

Table 6.3
Level 2 assessment of
Fiona Starr

Assessment Level 1 – Behaviour	Assessment Level 2 – Stimuli		
	Focal	Contextual	Residual
a(i)*	Odour Lymphoedema Fungation	Nursed away from other patients Dressing not suited to wound	May have previous experience of seeing dying patients with wounds
a(ii)	Frequent dressing changes	Nurses' attitude when performing dressing changes	Previous information given about progress of wound
b(i)	Children and husband upset at Fiona's condition	Hospice setting and attitude of staff to Fiona	Information given at previous treatment consultations

* See Table 6.2.

PRACTICE POINTS

- The management of the wound must focus around the stimuli causing Fiona's particular behaviour.
- Fiona needs counselling to adapt her behaviour to a more balanced view to help her and her family cope.
- She needs to talk through her treatment decisions and come to terms with why she made the decision she did.
- What particular wound management could she have that would help her to adapt?

FACTITIOUS WOUNDS

Factitious or self-inflicted wounds can pose enormous problems to health-care staff, as shown in Case study 6.5.

Case study 6.5

Self-inflicted injury

Justina Finlay has presented to her general practitioner with an area of necrotic tissue above the inside of her left ankle.

On examination, the wound is 4 cm in diameter with a surrounding area of inflamed tissue. The general practitioner does not know Justina very well but takes only a brief history and sends her to the practice nurse for a dressing.

Justina does not go into the practice nurse's treatment room that day but presents herself three days later in a somewhat anxious state. Sister Andrews, an experienced nurse who has worked both in general nursing and psychiatry, sits Justina down and, before looking at her wound, spends some time asking her about her medical and social history.

Justina is unemployed and lives in a small caravan with some friends on the outskirts of the town. She states that she cut her ankle while chopping wood and had tried to dress it herself but that it has gone septic-looking and now black.

Examination of the wound revealed widespread cellulitis and phlebitis surrounding an obviously infected, necrotic wound (Figure 6.13). Sister Andrews attempted mechanical debridement of the wound but this was too painful and Justina became agitated and threatened to leave the surgery. The nurse measured Justina's temperature (which was 39.5°C) and blood pressure; while doing so she noticed needle marks covering the arm.

Figure 6.13
Justina Finlay's ankle showing self-inflicted wound following assumed intravenous drug abuse.

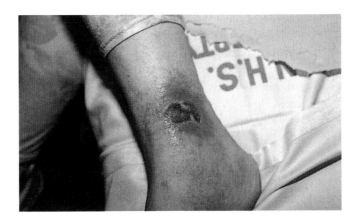

Aetiology   It is a common assumption by clinicians that the shared goal or outcome for both the patient with a wound and the professionals caring for that patient is to achieve healing of the wound (Baragwanath et al 1994a). However, for a small percentage of patients this is not the case and individuals may be responsible for either creating a wound or preventing an existing wound from healing.

More than 24 000 teenagers are admitted annually to hospital after deliberately harming themselves and around 1 in 10 self-harm (Department of Health 2004). These rates are among the highest in Europe but may be even higher as many cases are treated at home (NICE 2004b). Young people who self-harm are trying to communicate how they feel inside and are having difficulties in doing so, and they often need professional help to achieve this (NICE 2004b). One study established the incidence of factitious wounds as being 0.5% of non-healing wounds attending a specialist wound clinic (Baragwanath et al 1994b). This study reported that although the mean age at which patients received treatment for their factitious wounds was 44 years, the mean age of onset of the wounds was much lower, at 34 years, with equal numbers of men and women presenting. Young patients had a particular set of social circumstances thought to be associated with their psychotic illness. All young people were single and still living at home with their parents. For this young group of patients the average age of onset of the non-healing wound was 20 years and these individuals demonstrated limited social maturity and found difficulties in forming personal relationships outside their family group. As this illness progresses the young individual becomes increasingly socially isolated and dependent on both family and health-care professionals. Should the true nature of the non-healing wound be suspected and the patient confronted, denial is likely to be rapidly followed by the patient seeking referral to another health-care professional (NICE 2002b).

Although tempting, direct confrontation is not an effective approach for young individuals with factitious wounds. An alternative approach has been put forward (Baragwanath et al 1994a) in which the nurse or doctor informs the patient that they know what might have caused the wound not to heal but also, at the same time, offers an alternative explanation. A new wound treatment is then prescribed and the patient is told that if this new treatment is not effective that self-inflicted injury will be confirmed. This approach is helpful by offering the patient the choice of either stopping interfering with the wound or accepting the opportunity to receive psychotherapy. It also avoids the patient transferring to another health-care professional for the cycle to be repeated.

Management

The long-term outcome for these young patients is poor, with many wounds staying unhealed for some time.

This is undoubtedly a very difficult aspect of care to manage. Accurate documentation of the patient and wound assessment is crucial. The experienced nurse may identify a situation in which the appearance of the wound and the history the patient gives do not correspond. The first line of management should be to exclude physical causes for non-healing, which are often difficult to detect, and to obtain as much information as possible from previous medical and nursing notes. Remember that the patient may have received treatment in other hospitals or other parts of the country. Systemic and local infections need to be promptly treated as serious illness could result from such infection.

Above all, the nurse's manner and approach to the young individual in these difficult circumstances need careful thought. It is important for the nurse not to judge the patient by their own standards and to appreciate the complex nature of factitious illness.

The use of dressings which require infrequent changes with the minimum of fuss take the focus away from the wound. Occlusive dressings, such as hydrocolloids, also prevent the transmission of bacteria from the environment to the wound bed and help prevent the patient interfering with the wound.

Nursing model for Justina

Look back over this young woman's history. What do you suspect may be the cause of her wound?

The obvious conclusion would be that she is an injecting drug abuser and has used her leg veins for access but unless Justina is prepared to give Sister Andrews this information, how can it be proved?

The important feature of this case will be the nurse–patient interaction so Sister Andrews can use the Riehl interaction model (Riehl-Sisca 1989). The key information to be collected is the patient's 'definition' of the situation; therefore the nurse must attempt to enter into the patient's world in order to understand her viewpoint. Riehl underplays the physiological systems as the determinants of patients' problems, emphasizing the importance of psychosocial aspects.

In the first stage of the assessment it is necessary to ascertain whether Justina is adopting an appropriate role for her situation.

- Assessment (Stage 1): is Justina adopting an appropriate role for her present situation? (no)
- Planning (Stage 2): what are her problems related to? Physical? (yes) Psychological? (yes) Sociological? (yes).

It is necessary to identify the problems (Table 6.4) and negotiate patient-centred goals (Table 6.5).

Table 6.4
Identification of Justina's
problems (Case study 6.5)

Psychological	Physical	Sociological
Denial of cause of wound (A)	Necrotic non-healing wound (A)	Involved in drug-taking subculture (A)
Barrier between nurse and patient (A)	Localized infection (A)	Not in long-term employment (A)
Requires help for wound but reluctant to seek it (A)	Invasive infection and septicaemia (P)	Lives in squalid housing conditions (A)
Stigma associated with type of wound (A)	Loss of use of foot/limb (P)	
Fear of drug problem being exposed (A)	Infection with HIV, AIDS (A or P) Addition to abusive substance (A)	

(A), actual problem; (P), potential problem.

PRACTICE POINTS

■ Justina belongs to a subculture where drug-taking is the norm and personal self-esteem is low.

■ Sister Andrews attempts to build a relationship with Justina by involving her in her care and seeking her opinion.

■ She realizes that Justina may not attend the surgery again, so attempts to teach her some kind of self-care but also liaises with the community nurses. Much of her care is a form of role play because she demonstrates to Justina that she is non-judgemental about her drug abuse but cares about her physical condition.

■ She cannot cure the drug problem but she provides opportunities for Justina to seek help if desired.

■ The wound may not heal, especially if Justina tries to gain access to a vein in the same site.

■ The overall aim of management, therefore, is not necessarily wound healing but to gain the patient's trust so that her real problem (drug abuse) can be dealt with.

Table 6.5
Patient-centred goals and interventions planned for Justina (Case study 6.5)

Goal	Intervention
Psychological Enable patient to reveal her problem of drug abuse by forming a trusting relationship between nurse and patient	i) Display a non-judgemental attitude to Justina when attending to the wound ii) Give ample opportunity for Justina to discuss her problems iii) Stress confidentiality of treatment and any patient details recorded iv) Ensure treatment time will be undisturbed by other members of the practice v) Indicate that you are aware of her problem, but will only discuss it if she wishes vi) Allow Justina to see her records – do not hide them from her
To form a trusting relationship between nurse and patient	i) Display a concerned attitude towards Justina's general physical and mental condition ii) Involve Justina in planning care for her wound, and seek her opinion iii) Explain the nature of wound healing and the risk of possible infection iv) Ensure Justina knows whom to contact if the condition of the wound deteriorates v) Encourage Justina to discuss her relationship with family and friends vi) Ensure that she is given correct information regarding the treatment plan
Physiological Removal of necrotic tissue to promote healing of wound	i) Cover wound with a hydrocolloid dressing to promote autolysis and provide a protective barrier ii) Take a wound swab to confirm the type of organisms present in the wound iii) Teach Justina safe methods of cleaning her wound and reapplying the dressing (role play) iv) Liaise with community nurses to arrange home visits v) Document size, site and appearance of wound on initial and subsequent visits
To prevent spread of infection systemically	i) Explain the importance of keeping the wound clean ii) Ensure use of gloves when removing and reapplying dressings iii) Doctor to prescribe course of prophylactic antibiotics iv) Explain importance of taking antibiotic cover v) Arrange a mutually convenient time for Justina to attend the surgery
Sociological To facilitate opportunities for Justina to improve her socio-economic status	i) Provide information regarding helplines, drug counsellors, etc. ii) Ensure Justina has appropriate benefit entitlement

SUMMARY

This chapter has reflected on five different examples of the range of situations encountered by young adults.

Mostly healing will take place in this age group without too many physiological complications; however, psychological and sociological problems will require as much if not more attention to ensure the patient reaches a satisfactory outcome.

The type of models used highlight the following important issues:

- the patient and nurse plan care together to meet the patient's needs
- the nurse can attempt to understand the problems from the patient's perspective
- the effect the wound will have on the patient's normal living patterns
- the range of available dressings that the patient can manage alone
- the nurse remains non-judgemental and uses her counselling skills to gain the patient's trust.

These are skills that are gained through clinical experience and reflective practice. Look for somebody in your clinical area who you feel possesses these skills and watch how they interact with their patients.

FURTHER READING

Dealey C 1999 The care of wounds. Blackwell Scientific, Oxford.

Eagle M 1993 The care of a patient after a caesarean section. Journal of Wound Care 2(6): 330–336.

Grocott P 1995 The palliative management of fungating malignant wounds. Journal of Wound Care 4(5): 240–242.

Mishtriki S K, Jeffery P J, Law D J W 1992 Wound infection: the surgeon's responsibility. Journal of Wound Care 1(2): 32–36.

Müller C, O'Neill A, Mortimer D 1993 Skin problems in palliative care: nursing aspects. In: Doyle D, Hanks G, McDonald N (eds) Oxford textbook of palliative medicine. Oxford Medical, Oxford.

REFERENCES

American Canoe Association 2004 Safety Report <http://www.acanet.org/>. Accessed 29.3.05.

Baragwanath P, Shutler S, Harding KG 1994a The management of a patient with a factitious wound. Journal of Wound Care 3(6): 286–287.

Baragwanath P, Gruffudd-Jones A, Young H L, Harding K G 1994b Factitious behaviour in the aetiology of non-healing wounds. Proceedings of the Fourth European Conference on Advances in Wound Management. Macmillan, London.

Bascom J U 1994 Pilonidal sinus. Current Practice in Surgery 6: 175–180.

Berry D P 1992 Pilonidal sinus disease. Journal of Wound Care 1(3): 29–32.

Coulter A 2000 More active role for patients. Nursing Standard 14(45): 5.

Cutting K F, White R J 2004 Criteria for wound infection by indication. In: White R J (ed) Trends in wound care, vol III. Quay Books, Salisbury.

Department of Health 1991 The NHS plan. HMSO, London.

Department of Health 2004 National suicide prevention strategy for England. London: Department of Health.

Duxbury M S, Blake S M, Dashfield A, Lambert A W 2003 A randomised trial of knife versus diathermy in pilonidal disease. Annals of Royal College of Surgeons of England 85: 405–407.

Gurney J G, Severson R K, Davis S, Robison L L 1995 Incidence of cancer in children in the United States. Cancer 75: 2186–2195.

Jones D J 1992 Pilonidal sinus. British Medical Journal 305: 410–412.

Khairi H S, Brown J H 1995 Excision and primary closure of pilonidal sinus. Annals of Royal College of Surgeons of England 77: 242–244.

Kitchen P R B 1996 Pilonidal sinus: experience with the Karydarkis flap. British Journal of Surgery 83: 1452–1455.

Kramarova E, Stiller C A 1996 The international classification of childhood cancer. International Journal of Cancer 68: 759–765.

Link M P, Eiler F 1997 Osteosarcoma. In: Pizzo P A, Poplack D G (eds) Principles and practices of pediatric oncology. Lippencott-Raven, Philadelphia, Pennsylvania.

McQueen A 2000 Nurse-patient relationships and partnerships in hospital care. Journal of Clinical Nursing 9(5): 723–731.

Miller D, Harding K 2003 Pilonidal sinus disease. World Wide Wounds. Available online at: www.worldwidewounds.com. Accessed 30.08.04.

Miller R W, Boice J D, Curtis R E 1996 Bone cancer. In: Schottenfield D, Fraumeni J F (eds) Cancer epidemiology and prevention. Oxford University Press, New York.

NICE 2004a Clinical guideline 13: caesarean section. Available online at: www.nice.org.uk/CGO13NICEguideline. Accessed 30.08.04.

NICE 2004b Clinical guideline 16: short term physical and psychological management and secondary prevention of self-harm in primary and secondary care. Available at www.nice.org.uk/.

Orem D 1995 Nursing – concepts of practice, 5th edn. Mosby Yearbook, St Louis, Missouri.

Peplau H 1952 Interpersonal relations in nursing. G P Putman, New York.

Peterson S, Koch R, Stelzner S 2002 Primary closure techniques in chronic pilonidal sinus. A survey of the results of different surgical approaches. Diseases of the Colon and Rectum 45: 1458–1467.

Riehl-Sisca J P 1989 The Riehl interaction model. In: Riehl-Sisca J P (ed) Conceptual models for nursing practice, 3rd edn. Appleton and Lange, Norwalk, Connecticut.

Rodgers S E 1999 The patient facing surgery. In: Alexander M F, Fawcett J N, Runciman P J (eds) Nursing practice. Churchill Livingstone, Edinburgh.

Roy C, Andrews H 1999 The Roy adaptation model, 2nd edn. Appleton and Lange, Stamford, Connecticut.

Senapati A, Cripps N P J 2000 Pilonidal sinus. In: Johnson C D, Taylor I (eds) Recent advances in surgery 23. Churchill Livingstone, Edinburgh.

Senapati A, Cripps N P J, Thompson M R 2000 Bascom's operation in the day-surgical management of symptomatic pilonidal sinus. British Journal of Surgery 87: 1067–1070.

Smitherman C 1981 Nursing actions for health promotion. F A Davis, Philadelphia, Pennsylvania.

Thomas J, Paranjothy S 2001 Royal College of Obstetricians and Gynaecologists Clinical Effectiveness Support Unit. National Sentinel Caesarean Section Audit Report. RCOG Press, London.

Wound care in the middle-aged individual

KEY ISSUES

This chapter outlines the wound problems encountered by the middle-aged individual.

Clinical Case Studies

Aetiology and management of the following:

■ Neuropathic foot ulcer in a man with diabetes mellitus
■ Postoperative care of a patient following a partial mastectomy and breast reconstruction
■ A patient undergoing abdominal perineal resection.

Nursing Models

Examples of their application to practice are taken from:

■ Peplau's model
■ Roy's adaptation model
■ Orem's model.

PRACTICE POINTS

As you read through this chapter concentrate on the following:

■ the effect of serious illness on a previously healthy adult
■ the nurse in an educative and supportive role
■ the use of specialist nurses to complement the care given to these patients
■ the importance that underlying disease processes have on wound healing.

INTRODUCTION

For many individuals the teenage and adult years are full of activity, parenting and hard work. Middle age can bring financial stability and contentment. When illness happens at this stage of the life-cycle patients can have difficulty accepting it. Malignancy, diabetes mellitus and cardiovascular disease are frequently encountered diseases for this age group.

DIABETIC FOOT ULCERATION

Diabetic foot ulcers are a serious complication of diabetes mellitus. The problem can be compounded by the patient's lifestyle, as in Case study 7.1.

Case study 7.1

Diabetic foot ulceration

Donald Waites has had insulin-dependent diabetes mellitus for 30 years, having been diagnosed at the age of 25 years. Following diagnosis of his condition, Donald was very careful in following the advice given and took his insulin according to his blood glucose levels. Patient education was sparse at that time as there were no specialist nurses or clinics and management was largely controlled by the hospital consultant or general practitioner. As time progressed, like many individuals with diabetes mellitus, Donald began to disregard advice and gave himself extra insulin when going out for a large meal and drinking heavily.

In his 30s and 40s he had many epsiodes of hypoglycaemia and hyperglycaemia, which on several occasions resulted in admission to hospital. Education regarding diet, weight control and foot care was reinforced on these occasions but by now Donald was becoming resistant to the advice of health professionals, feeling that he had received little support in coping with his condition over the years. These periods of hospitalization resulted in Donald's employment becoming sporadic and he often found himself without work and having to claim unemployment benefit in order to support himself.

At present Donald, now 55 years old, is working on a building site as a bricklayer. He is single and has no dependants. Working long hours to claim overtime, he continues to bypass regular meals or insulin. His personal hygiene has also deteriorated and his housing conditions are squalid.

As far as diabetic management goes, he has not visited his general practitioner for the last two years, even though he has been experiencing 'pins and needles' in his arms and hands and a loss of sensation in both feet. This has frightened Donald as at this time of his life he is fearful of not having employment and being unable to draw a pension.

On return from work yesterday Donald took off his boot and found he had a round ulcer on his right heel. The skin surrounding the wound was red and inflamed and although he could feel nothing, he realized it had been caused by a nail sticking through the heel of his boot. Donald remembered a patient in the bed next to him during his last hospital visit who had had a similar ulcer, and also remembered that this man ended up having his leg amputated. Donald went to his doctor the very next morning.

Epidemiology and aetiology

Diabetic foot problems are the cause of more inpatient stays than all the other medical problems caused by diabetes (Frykberg 1999). The impact of foot ulceration on the individual's life is great, with the potential for amputation ever present. Diabetes is one of the most common endocrine diseases across all populations and age groups (Mandrup-Poulsen 1998), with insulin-dependent diabetes mellitus (IDDM) usually developing in childhood. Although most common in European populations, diabetes is on the increase worldwide (Rees & Gibby 1997). Williams (1995) has estimated that in the UK there are around

Figure 7.1
A neuropathic foot ulcer showing Charcot joints of the foot.

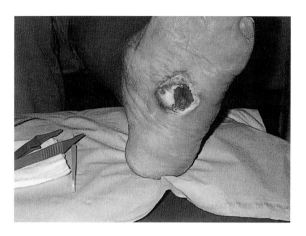

750 000 patients with diabetes mellitus. Of this group, 4% will have had an amputation, with a further 6% experiencing foot ulceration. This translates into around 30 000 patients either missing a limb or part of a limb, and 45 000 patients currently having foot ulceration.

Defined as a group of syndromes in which neuropathy, ischaemia and infection lead to tissue breakdown, both peripheral neuropathy and peripheral vascular disease can occur simultaneously. Infection is not a primary cause of ulceration but is a secondary complication and when present can lead to soft tissue necrosis and damage to underlying tendon and bone, possibly leading to amputation (World Health Organization 1999). The prevalence of both neuropathy and peripheral vascular disease increases with the duration of the diabetic condition. Below the age of 40 years foot ulceration is uncommon. Around 6% of diabetic patients aged 60–69 years experience foot ulceration, rising to 14% in those patients aged 80 years and over (Walters et al 1992). The nerve damage caused by diabetic neuropathy is generally thought to be the result of the accumulation of glucose metabolites, which cause osmotic swelling and damage to nerve cells (Pickup & Williams 1997).

■ Peripheral neuropathy: neuropathic ulcers are by far the most common cause of diabetic foot ulceration and are a serious complication of diabetes (Figure 7.1). Most commonly peripheral neuropathy affects the lower limbs and can affect sensory, motor or cutaneous nerves. Sensory impairment means that painless neuropathic ulcers can be caused by repeated pressure and trauma from ill-fitting shoes. Thermal trauma may be caused by the heat of fires or hot-water bottles, which the patient fails to feel. Chemical trauma may result from the diabetic patient applying home remedies, such as over-the-counter treatment for corns, instead of consulting a chiropodist. Patients with neuropathy may cut their toenails too harshly, get sunburnt feet or step on a sharp object without realizing that damage is being done.

■ Peripheral vascular disease: vascular insufficiency affects both large (atherosclerosis) and small vessels (microvascular disease) of the lower limbs (Jeffcoate & Harding 2003). The distal cells are deprived of the necessary metabolic requirements and the tissues become devitalized. Subsequent injury from ill-fitting footwear can then readily cause **ischaemic** ulceration of the area (Figure 7.2).

Figure 7.2
Patient with peripheral vascular disease due to diabetes. The great and first toe have already been amputated due to gangrene.

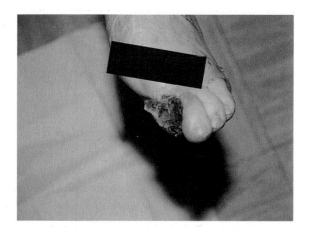

Thrombosis can also occur, resulting in gangrene of the area supplied by the thrombosed vessel. So, gangrene can result from a seemingly minor injury, with very serious consequences. Both life and limb are at risk in this situation. The affected limb, or part of the limb, may require amputation, with infection and septicaemia being potentially lethal.

Identifying the patient at risk of developing foot ulceration is essential if ulceration is to be prevented or damage minimized. The production of the SIGN guidelines in 2001 identified risk factors for diabetic patients as those shown in Box 7.1.

Many diabetic foot problems can be prevented or the damage minimized through careful monitoring of the patient's feet. Protective measures are listed in Box 7.2.

Box 7.1 Risk factors for developing ulceration or gangrene (from SIGN 2001)

1. Previous ulceration or gangrene
2. Increasing age
3. Peripheral vascular disease
4. Neuropathy
5. Joint deformity
6. Presence of callus
7. Other:
    duration of diabetes
    male sex
    retinopathy
    nephropathy
    visual/mobility problems

Assessment and diagnosis

A full history and examination should be performed relating to the patient's diabetes. If this has already been done, accurate documentation should be obtained of the previous history.

Box 7.2 Measures to protect the feet in diabetes mellitus (from CREST 1998)

General measures
- Do not smoke
- Take a varied and balanced diet to promote good glycaemic control and wound healing
- Exercise. Try to keep active. This will help both neuropathy and ischaemia

Basic footcare advice
- Try to get shoes which don't pinch anywhere and which allow all toes to move freely. New shoes should never need to be broken in
- Ensure that socks or stockings fit comfortably. Change them daily
- Change footwear as soon as possible if wet
- Avoid walking barefoot; wear slippers and beach shoes to prevent injury
- Bathe feet daily using lukewarm (not hot) water and mild soap
- Pat feet dry gently; pay special attention to the area between the toes
- Apply a moisturizing cream daily (except between the toes) to avoid dryness and keep the skin supple
- Avoid exposing feet to excess heat or cold
- Cut nails to the shape of the end of the toe
- Do not self-treat corns and calluses
- If a minor cut or abrasion does occur, wash thoroughly and cover with a sterile dressing. Seek advice if it has not healed within a few days

Specific advice for patients with neuropathy/ischaemia
- Inspect feet daily for blisters, corns, calluses, cracks or redness (a mirror can help in seeing the underside of the foot)
- Use of footwear when walking
- Check shoes and socks before putting them on
- Access the foot care service
- Seek advice for treatment of callus from podiatrist
- Learn the warning signs of infection and other foot problems

---

Central to the diagnosis is an integrated clinical examination of the foot (Figure 7.3). Assessment should aim to:

- ascertain the type, onset and duration of diabetes
- identify current or developing complications of diabetes
- diagnose the exact nature and aetiology of the ulcer
- prescribe the correct medical or surgical treatment
- identify suitable dressing and foot care that will enhance healing.

Important points to be recorded are summarized in Table 7.1, while Table 7.2 lists the clinical features that differentiate neuropathic and ischaemic ulceration.

Figure 7.3
Neuropathic ulcers of both feet. These wounds require debridement of necrotic tissue and callus before wound assessment can take place.

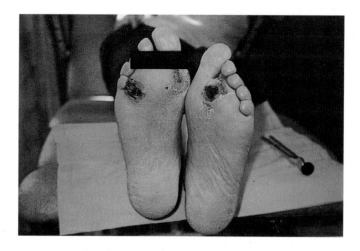

Table 7.1
Important facts to be ascertained in patients with diabetic ulceration (reproduced with kind permission from Harding & Jones 1996)

Record	Rationale
Date of birth	Age is a risk factor for PVD
Sex	PVD and amputations more common in men
Type of diabetes and treatment	Methods of achieving good control. May change treatment if control poor
Duration of diabetes	Prevalence of neuropathy and ischaemia increase with duration
History of ischaemic heart disease, myocardial infarctions, cerebrovascular accident, angina	Indication of arteriosclerosis and ischaemia
Smoking	Risk factor for PVD in diabetic patients
Compliance	Key factor in aetiology of ulcer and aftercare management
History of intermittent claudication	Indicative of ischaemia
Rest pain	
Previous arterial surgery	
PVD, peripheral vascular disease	

Specific examinations

For ischaemia Palpation of pedal pulses is not a reliable indicator for the assessment of ischaemia and should not be used (Moffatt & O'Hare 1995). Doppler assessment and measurement of ankle brachial pressure index (see Chapter 9) will indicate an ischaemic cause for the ulceration. The Doppler ultrasound reading can be used in conjunction with clinical examination to confirm the presence of ischaemia. Patients with diabetes mellitus may give falsely high (i.e. normal) readings owing to calcification of the arteries so they should always be viewed with caution and in conjunction with a full medical history. In specialist units other more in-depth vascular assessments may be carried out such as transcutaneous oxygen tension (TcPO$_2$) and plethysmography.

Table 7.2
Differential diagnosis of neuropathic and ischaemic ulceration

Clinical feature	Neuropathic foot	Ischaemic foot
Colour	Normal or red appearance indicating cellulitis or early Charcot foot	Pale/cyanotic Rubor on dependency Blanches on elevation (Buerger's test)
Deformity	Claw toe Hammer toe Charcot deformity	Nil Absent toes from previous surgery
Callus tissue	Found on plantar surface of metatarsal head/apices or toes	Nil – thin skin
Tissue breakdown	Ulcers commonly found on plantar surface	Ulcers commonly found on the margins Visible signs of digital gangrene
Peripheral pulses	Present (may be difficult to palpate if swollen or deformed foot)	Dorsalis pedis and/or posterior tibial absent May not be absent if small vessel disease
Temperature	Feels normal or warm	Feels cold
Skin moisture	Dry foot Decrease in perspiration	Normal
Sensation	Impaired sensation to pinprick/light touch position and vibration	Normal
Tendon reflex	Impaired	Normal

Reproduced with kind permission from Harding & Jones (1996).

Table 7.3
Other investigations in diabetic foot ulceration

Record	Rationale
Haemoglobin HbA1c	Good measure of long-term control
Urea and creatinine	Measurement of renal function indicative of nephropathy
Proteinuria	Indicative of nephropathy
Wound swab	Confirms clinical signs of infection

For neuropathy The vibration threshold can be measured using a biothesiometer; vibrations can be transmitted through the patient's foot to indicate the extent of sensory loss. Simpler measurements using a 128 Hz tuning fork or a 10 g Semmes-Weinstein monofilament can be performed by any practitioner.

Other examinations Retinal examination indicates the absence or degree of retinopathy. Other investigations are listed in Table 7.3.

Management Healing is likely to be impaired in the patient with diabetes mellitus as there is a reduction in the inflammatory response and granulation tissue formation. Neuropathic ulcers usually take weeks or months to heal, even with the appropriate resources. Some patients require complete bed rest combined with removal of weight bearing and friction. For patients with ischaemic ulcers, reconstructive arterial surgery should always be considered, although the optimum time for this to happen is difficult to judge (SIGN 2001). Generally patients with neuropathic ulcers will have the best healing times but an overall rate of 62% has been achieved in ulcers of mixed disease (Abelqvist et al 1993).

- General issues related to the disease process of diabetes mellitus should be considered, i.e. control of the disease and referral to the appropriate specialist for reconstructive surgery or medical treatment of complications.
- Continuing care and maintenance of the foot can be given, ideally at a multidisciplinary foot clinic or by a chiropodist/podiatrist. Nail and foot care can be provided and problems detected at an early stage.
- Ideally all weight should be relieved from the ulcerated area and redistributed. This can be achieved by an orthotist designing and making footwear for the patient.
- Daily inspection of the feet by the patient should be undertaken, regardless of whether the foot is ulcerated or not. Any signs of redness, heat, blistering or bleeding should be looked for and immediate treatment sought. If ignored, the foot could rapidly deteriorate and lead to invasive infection of the limb.
- Dressings useful for the treatment of foot ulceration include absorbent foams which act as padding and protection for the injured area. For moderate or heavily exuding ulcers, alginate dressings can provide absorbency without too much bulk. Semiocclusive dressings such as hydrocolloids or adhesive dressings which are not changed daily and so prevent daily foot inspection are best avoided.
- Regular debridement of callus build-up around the ulcer bed is advised. All callus, or as much as possible, should be removed to prevent further trauma to the area.
- Patient education is of paramount importance in the prevention and/or deterioration of foot ulcers. Education will help to empower the patient to take control of their condition and minimize complications (Meetoo 2004).

Nursing model for Donald

Having visited his general practitioner, who performed a full assessment (see Table 7.4), Donald was diagnosed as having a neuropathic foot ulcer.

The general practitioner transferred wound care to the district nurse. If the district nurse uses Peplau's model, what particular aspects of the model are pertinent to assessing and planning Donald's care?

Development models often focus on the educative-counselling role the nurse plays. This is of paramount importance, as often the care a patient needs may be different from what they want. Do you think that Donald wants the care and advice the district nurse is going to give? (Probably he does not.)

Peplau's philosophy of nursing stresses the importance of the formation of the relationship between nurse and patient. The first purpose of the nurse is to minimize or remove the risks to the patient's health but the second is to help the individual to understand and come to terms with their health problem. In Donald's case this will require a great deal of input.

Table 7.4
Assessment of Donald's problems (Case study 7.1)

Subjective experience of patient	Objective observation by nurse
Little faith in health professionals	Patient non-compliant with treatment
Not wanting to be labelled as ill	Patient unaware of health status
Feels he can control illness by altering insulin according to social needs	Little understanding of the pathology of the disease process
Frightened of the consequences of his complaint	Has not reported signs of neuropathy until ulcer developed Displaying signs of advanced disease process
Frightened that ulceration could lead to amputation	Localized infection in and around ulcer, possibility of invasive infection
Does not understand why he did not feel nail in shoe rubbing	Not aware of signs of diabetic neuropathy Does not inspect feet daily
Finds it increasingly difficult to keep up with personal hygiene and domestic chores	Looks unkempt; nobody at home to provide support
Worried that period of sickness will result in unemployment	Financial difficulties due to sporadic employment

Table 7.5
Identification of problems in Table 7.4 and plan of action

Identification of problem	Plan of action
Infected neuropathic ulcer	Debridement of ulcer by doctor, nurse or chiropodist Daily dressing with absorbent dressing (foam or alginate), wound cleansing with saline to remove dressing material Swab to identify infecting organism, treat with broad-spectrum antibiotic orally initially One-week period of non-weight bearing
Poor understanding of diet and diabetic control	Diabetic specialist nurse and community dietician to visit patient at home District nurse to reinforce information with patient education programme
Long-term history of unstable diabetes	Assessment of HbAc blood test Renal function, eye retinopathy, extent of neuropathy Referral to diabetic specialist
Lack of knowledge concerning care of feet	District nurse to explain importance of inspection of feet daily, hygiene and clean footwear Refer to orthotist for removal of friction Refer to chiropodist
Reluctant to seek support of health professionals	District nurse to promote a trusting relationship with patient by listening to his point of view Planning care together with realistic goals Introducing other specialists to patients at separate intervals
Lives alone, no social support	Encourage patient to joint local diabetic association; find out details of local group
Fear of loss of employment and lack of secure income	Arrange visit of social worker to reassess benefit entitlement Consider change of employment to less manual work

PRACTICE POINT Donald Waites' case stresses the importance of the nurse's role in helping patients to understand and come to terms with their condition.

Look at Tables 7.4 and 7.5, compiled using the SOAP acronym (S, subjective experience of patient; O, objective observation made by nurse; A, assessment and identification of problems on S and O; P, plan of action).

BREAST CANCER *Case study 7.2 outlines the case of a woman who has undergone a partial mastectomy for removal of a breast tumour.*

Case study 7.2 **Partial mastectomy and breast reconstruction**
Mrs Joyce Harris is recovering in hospital following a partial mastectomy and breast reconstruction. The operation to remove a tumour from her left breast was performed four days ago. She now has two transverse suture lines, one across the reconstructed left breast, the other across her abdomen from which tissue was taken to perform the reconstructive surgery.

Joyce, who is 46 years old, is progressing well and is pleased with the cosmetic results of her breast. She has been informed that all the tumour was removed but will require a few weeks of radiotherapy as a precaution.

The suture lines are clean and non-inflamed.

Epidemiology and aetiology

In the UK around 11 500 women die as a result of breast cancer, which is the most common form of cancer affecting women. In 2000 there were almost 36 000 new cases and one in nine women will develop breast cancer at some point in their lives (Office for National Statistics 2003). Risk factors relate to early first period, late first pregnancy, late menopause and hereditary causes such as family history of breast cancer.

Breast cancers arise from the epithelial cells within the terminal duct lobular unit of the breast. Cancer cells will either remain within the terminal duct lobular unit and the draining duct (in situ or non-invasive) or disseminate out into the surrounding tissue and beyond (invasive) (Salisbury et al 2000).

- In situ/non-invasive: the malignant cells are contained within the originating tissue and have not spread outwards into surrounding tissues, the cancer remains in situ within the tissue of origin.
- Invasive: the malignant cells have spread into the surrounding tissues.
- Differentiation: the malignant cells are histologically described as being poorly, moderately or well differentiated. Well-differentiated malignant cells closely resemble the tissue in which they originated. They are less aggressive than poorly differentiated cells, which metastasize (spread to distant sites) at an early stage.

Tumour differentiation can be scored and graded and will be a useful predictor of the type of treatment offered, local recurrence and the overall prognosis for the patient

Diagnosis

Following the discovery of a lump or mass in the breast or detection of a mass on mammography, the woman will be referred to a breast specialist centre. It is likely that a number of investigations will be performed at this early stage. A full medical history will be taken by the breast specialist, which is followed by a physical examination including clinical examination of the breast. The woman will almost certainly be extremely anxious and concerned about her well-being and would be best advised for this crucial hospital visit to be accompanied by her partner or a friend. Other investigations carried out at this time may include a mammogram, fine-needle aspiration of the mass or lump for cytology (FNAC), ultrasonography to differentiate between lumps and cysts, and in some cases excisional biopsy for the diagnosis of lymph node metastasis (Roth 1999). It will take several days for the results of these types of investigation to be reported and for the breast specialist to make a firm diagnosis. This is an extremely stressful time for the woman and her family.

A range of treatment options are now available from surgery, radiotherapy, chemotherapy and other adujvant therapies such as hormone therapy. Surgery may range from simple excision of the breast lump to a wide local excision of the lump, partial or segmental mastectomy or simple mastectomy possibly with axillary dissection of lymph glands (Dixon 2002). Radiotherapy and chemotherapy may be offered in addition to surgery. All postmenopausal women are offered an oestrogen-blocking drug, tamoxifen, as an adjuvant therapy. Postmenopausal women have high levels of oestrogen receptors and this drug works by blocking the oestrogen from stimulating cancer cell growth (Early Breast Cancer Trialists Group 1998).

Incidence rates of breast cancer have increased but with earlier detection and improved treatment, survival rates year on year have risen. Death rates have fallen and survival from breast cancer is better than that for cancer of the cervix (Office for National Statistics 2003).

Postoperative care

The suture lines need to be observed for signs of clinical infection and this observation linked to measurements of temperature and pulse. The primary wound dressing can be left undisturbed if a transparent dressing has been used and only changed if it becomes too soiled. It is also usual for low-suction drainage to be used; one drain is inserted under the suture lines and another in the axillary area, both sites where haematoma formation is likely. After 48 hours these may be removed when the drainage subsides.

Nursing model for Joyce

Joyce requires basic postoperative care for her wounds. The surgery has been elective and at a site with a low risk of contamination. However, think of the wider implications of this type of surgery and the cosmetic and psychological effects this type of wound has on any woman.

Table 7.6
Application of Roy's assessment model to the problems of Mrs Harris (Case study 7.2)

Life Area	Assessment Level 1 – Behaviour	Assessment Level 2 – Stimuli		
		Focal	Contextual	Residual
Physiological Rest and activity	Unable to move arm and sit up straight	Wound painful		Fear of splitting stitches
Regulation	Pain in breast and abdomen	Surgery, anxiety	Afraid to bother nurses for pain relief	Afraid to take too many pain-killers
	Wound dehiscence Wound infection	No obvious signs	Wound breakdown likely at 10 days	
Self-concept	Worried about scarring	Wound sutured	Underlying malignancy may retard healing	Has heard bad reports of breast reconstruction
	Loss of 'normal' body appearance	Left breast shape different from right	Final shape may differ	Breast shape not as shown in pictures of reconstruction
	Fear of recurrence of disease	Only lump removed, not whole breast	Doctors cannot give 100% assurance	Has no experience of others with same problem
Role function	Loss of femininity	Sutured wounds ugly	Feels tired and depressed after operation	
	Loss of role as husband's sexual partner	Husband's anxiety has changed his manner with her		

Joyce needs to adapt to her new body image and may perceive that she has lost her sexual attractiveness; maybe Roy's adaptation model would be a good choice here (Table 7.6).

PRACTICE POINTS

■ By assessing the focal, contextual or residual origins of the various problems, the nurse can plan appropriate interventions.

■ What are the major features required to give Joyce optimum care? Wound care may not be the most important issue in this case. The services of the specialist breast nurse should be enlisted to provide support and advice to this patient.

COLORECTAL CANCER

Case study 7.3 illustrates the problems that may follow an abdominoperineal resection for colorectal cancer.

Case study 7.3

Abdominoperineal resection

Harold Mathews is a 62-year-old man, a widower for 10 years, who runs a large dairy farm with his two sons.

For some time, he had experienced problems with a change in his bowel habit and eventually was persuaded by his elder son to go and see his doctor.

Harold was admitted to hospital for tests and diagnosed as having an adenocarcinoma of the rectum. An abdominoperineal resection was performed within a matter of days following diagnosis, leaving Harold with a colostomy, a sutured laparotomy line and a perineal wound left open to heal by secondary intention. Harold was determined to recover quickly as he was not used to hospital and disliked people fussing over him.

Preoperatively Harold was visited by the stomatherapist who helped him decide where to site his stoma and which appliances to use. During the postoperative period Harold quickly mastered changing the colostomy bags and gained confidence. His laparotomy wound healed well and sutures were removed 10 days postoperatively.

Harold's perineal wound measured 6 cm long, 3 cm wide and 8 cm deep on discharge from hospital. Granulation tissue had covered the wound bed which was healthy and clean. In hospital the wound had been irrigated daily while the patient was taking a shower and the ward nurses had taken considerable care to treat this as part of his daily hygiene. Once Harold had dried after showering, an absorbent pad protected his clean pyjamas until he returned to his bed for a dressing renewal. The perineal wound was inspected carefully at these daily dressing changes, the nurses looking for pocketing and tracking in the depths of the wound, and wound measurements were taken weekly. The wound was packed with an alginate rope which Harold found comfortable and absorbent.

He was discharged home after 10 days in hospital, to the care of the district nurse who would look after his perineal wound on a daily basis using alginate and monitor his progress. On his first evening home Harold appeared to lose all confidence and panicked. His younger son, who still lives on the farm, found him in the early hours of the morning in the bathroom crying because his stoma bag had come loose during the night and had soiled his pyjamas. The district nurse was due to call that day.

Aetiology

Colorectal cancer is the third most common malignancy in the United Kingdom, most often occurring in people in later life in their 60s and 70s. Although there appeared to be a prevalence in men (Burkitt 1971), latest figures reveal that it affects men and women almost equally (Cancer Research 2003). The cause of colorectal cancer is difficult to determine but it has been linked to the low-residue diet and lifestyle of the affluent populations (Burkitt 1971). However, most colorectal cancers result from malignant changes to adenomas (polyps) which develop naturally in about 20% of the population. A small number will inherit a gene disorder and tend to develop bowel cancer before the age of 50 (Scholefield 2000).

The onset of the disease is often gradual and it is not unusual for patients to present to their general practitioner only when the disease is at an advanced stage. Patients experience vague symptoms of a gradual change of bowel habit, with constipation alternating with diarrhoea. It takes 10–15 years for a pre-malignant adenoma to develop into carcinoma but outcome for the patient is markedly improved with early detection from colorectal screening that has targeted the 55–65 year group (Scholefield 2000).

Management

Middle-aged and elderly individuals are often reluctant to present to their doctor with symptoms related to colorectal disease. Education about bowel cancer is poor, with large numbers of the general population unaware that cancer of the bowel can occur (Young et al 1996). Very often the onset of colorectal cancer is gradual and vague, often without pain until the cancer obstructs or partially obstructs the colon. Patients can easily mistake bleeding and mucus in the stool for haemorrhoids, with changes in bowel habit being related to problems with food. It is common for patients to present with bowel obstruction and acute abdominal pain. Emergency surgery is likely to result in the tumour being excised together with the rectum and the formation of a permanent colostomy. There is often little time to prepare the patient for this extensive, disfiguring surgery. Around 100 000 people in the UK have a stoma of some type, be that colostomy, ileostomy or urostomy. Of these, some 30 000 have a permanent colostomy and around 6500 patients a year have a permanent colostomy formed (Liles 1995). Many patients experience extreme trauma following formation of a permanent colostomy. Body image is severely altered, leading to anxiety, loss of confidence, rejection, social isolation, depression and sexual dysfunction. Patients with a colostomy can find that their lifestyle is changed beyond recognition in the initial months following surgery, owing to the loss of control of their bowel habits and the struggle to gain control of the stoma (Black 2000).

The help of a specialist stoma nurse preoperatively where possible and also in the postoperative period is invaluable in providing both counselling and practical help and advice. Patients should have the opportunity to choose the stoma appliance most suited to their lifestyle. This is a stressful time for patients; having to accept a permanent stoma is difficult when recovering from unexpected major surgery.

Deep perineal wounds require careful observation and dressing. Assessments and measurements weekly should demonstrate steady progress towards healing, with evidence that the wound is healing from its depths with reduction in both depth and width as wound contraction takes place. Gentle examination of the wound should exclude pocketing and premature bridging in the depths of the wound. The professional help and support initiated in hospital in the immediate postoperative phase will need to be continued once the patient has returned home.

Nursing model for Harold

Think about the type of person Harold is before planning his care. A farmer all his life, still very active in the running of his farm, he is used to looking after himself since widowed.

He needs a long period of recuperation and support from those providing care but probably needs to regain as much independence as possible. It often happens that patients in hospital feel confident and appear on the surface to be coming to terms with their surgery. A large operation such as this requires long-term management.

Using Orem's model, we can assess Harold's deficits. The district nurse should, of course, decide whether these deficits are due to lack of knowledge, skill or motivation or limited range of behaviour (Table 7.7). Can you identify his self-care deficits?

PRACTICE POINTS

This type of situation is not uncommon. Patients often feel alone and fearful following discharge from the security of the hospital.

- The district nurse will need to gain Harold's confidence but also should enlist the support of specialist nurses and other primary care team members to help him recover a normal social pattern.
- His feelings are similar to those experienced when he lost his wife and the nurse must be aware of this.
- A plan of care must take into account his previous pattern of work on the farm as much as possible. This should include minimum dressing changes, using one that will remain in situ.

SUMMARY

Throughout this chapter there are two fundamental aspects that need to be addressed in order to provide a high level of wound care for an individual in this age group.

- The transition from health to *serious* illness in an adult requires the nurse to function in an educative role.
- All these cases require the input of specialist nurses who, with their expert skills, give a high level of professional care to their patients.

If you work with any specialist practitioners, observe the skills they use to enhance patient care.

Table 7.7
Self-care deficits for Harold Mathews (Case study 7.3)

Normal self-care ability (prior to operation)	Current self-care ability (following discharge home)	Self-care deficit (lack of knowledge, skill, motivation or limited behaviour)
Fluid balance Likes to drink beer (usually 2–3 pints at the weekend) Drinks large quantities of tea while working on farm	Rather dehydrated following operation, felt nauseous for some days, finds he does not have a 'taste' for drinks	
Nutrition Eats cooked breakfast and large cooked evening meal Lots of meat and vegetables	Loss of weight due to disease Does not feel like eating and worried about effect on colostomy	
Activity and rest Up at 5.30 every morning, works most of day until 8 at night Always active	Weak following surgery Wants to do things but cannot, feels frustrated and angry	
Socialization Lives with son since wife died 10 years ago Eats together with other son and daughter-in-law every Sunday Socializes in pub at weekends, at church on Sunday	Depressed and embarrassed about colostomy Worried he will smell when in church or having lunch Does not want sons to know about the bag	
Hazards Worries that once his son leaves he will be unable to manage farm and farmhouse	Worried about sons coping without him Long-term worries about how he will manage if son goes, now he has been so ill	
Normalcy Misses his wife greatly, as she helped on the farm as well as in the house	Has no-one to confide in and care for him Has managed to cope since his wife died, but feels out of control Does not want a nurse coming to the farm	
Health previously Never had reason to go to doctor Always uses local remedy to treat himself	Worried about the care of an open wound on farm Feels invalided and old Feels surgery was drastic and disease could have taken its course Does not know if he can resume normal work pattern	

FURTHER READING

Elkeles R S, Wolfe J H N 1993 The diabetic foot. ABC of vascular disease. British Medical Journal 303: 1053–1055.

Jeffcoate W, Macfarlane R 1996 The diabetic foot: an illustrated guide to management. Chapman and Hall Medical, London.

Malata C M, Williams N W, Shape D T 1995 Tissue expansion: an overview. Journal of Wound Care 4(1): 37–43.

Meeker M H, Rothrock J C (eds) 1999 Alexander's care of the patient in surgery, 11th edn. Mosby, Boston, Massachusetts.

REFERENCES

Abelqvist J, Larsson J, Agardh C-D 1993 Long term prognosis for diabetic patients with foot ulcers. Journal of Internal Medicine 233: 485–491.

Black P 2000 Practical stoma care. Nursing Standard 14(4): 47–53.

Burkitt D P 1971 Epidemiology of cancer of the colon and rectum. Cancer 28: 3–13.

Cancer Research 2003 Cancer stats. Cancer Research, London.

CREST 1998 Guidelines for wound management in Northern Ireland: guidelines for the management of the diabetic foot. Clinical Resource Efficiency Support Team, Belfast.

Dixon J M 2002 ABC of breast diseases, 2nd edn. BMJ Books, London.

Early Breast Cancer Trialists Collaborative Group 1998 Tamoxifen for early breast cancer: an overview of the randomised trials. Lancet 351: 1451–1467.

Frykberg R G 1999 Epidemiology of the diabetic foot: ulcerations and amputations. Advances in Wound Care 12(3): 139–141.

Harding K, Jones V 1996 Wound management: good practice guidance. Macmillan Magazines, London.

Jeffcoate W J, Harding K G 2003 Diabetic foot ulcers. Lancet 361: 1545–1551.

Liles L 1995 Stoma appliances: choices, prescription and problems. Prescriber Jan 5: 17–22.

Mandrup-Poulson T 1998 Diabetes – clinical review. British Medical Journal 316: 1221–1225.

Meetoo D 2004 Clinical skills: empowering people with diabetes to minimise complications. British Journal of Nursing 13(11): 644–651.

Moffatt C, O'Hare L 1995 Ankle pulses are not sufficient to detect impaired arterial circulation in patients with leg ulcers. Journal of Wound Care 4(3): 134–137.

Office for National Statistics 2003 National statistics. Available online at: www.statistics.gov.uk.

Pickup J C, Williams G (eds) 1997 The textbook of diabetes. 2nd edn. Blackwell Science, Oxford.

Rees D A, Gibby O M 1997 Diabetes: the nature of the disease. Journal of Wound Care Resource Pack.

Roth R A 1999 Breast surgery. In: Meeker M H, Rothrock J C (eds) Alexander's care of the patient in surgery, 11th edn. Mosby, Boston, Massachusetts.

Salisbury J R C, Anderson T J, Morgan D A 2000 ABC of breast diseases: breast cancer. British Medical Journal 321: 745–750.

Scholefield J H 2000 Screening: ABC of colorectal cancer. British Medical Journal 321: 1004–1006.

SIGN (2001) Management of diabetes: guideline 55. Scottish Intercollegiate Guidelines Network, Edinburgh.

Walters D P, Gatling W, Mullee M A, Hill R D 1992 The distribution and severity of diabetic foot disease: a community study with comparison to a non-diabetic group. Diabetic Medicine 9: 354–358.

Williams D R R 1995 The size of the problem: epidemiological and economic aspects of feet problems in diabetes. In: Boulton A J M, Connor H, Cavanagh P R (eds) The foot in diabetes, 2nd edn. John Wiley, Chichester.

World Health Organization 1999 Definition, diagnosis and classification of diabetes mellitus and its complications. Report of WHO consultation part 1: diagnosis and classification of diabetes mellitus. WHO, Geneva.

Young G P, Rozen P, Levin B (eds) 1996 Prevention and early detection of colorectal cancer. W B Saunders, London.

CHAPTER 8

Wound care in the elderly individual with a pressure ulcer

KEY ISSUES This chapter deals with the particular problems associated with wound healing in the elderly individual.

Clinical Case Study
- The aetiology and management of a patient with a pressure ulcer cared for in a nursing home.

Nursing Model
- Roper's model is used as an example of its application to practice.

PRACTICE POINTS As you read through this chapter concentrate on the following:

- recognition of the predisposing factors that contribute to pressure ulcer development
- use of the appropriate risk assessment tool to assess patients at risk
- thorough assessment of the pressure ulcer to ensure appropriate wound management
- involvement of the multidisciplinary team in delivery of care
- use of appropriate equipment to meet individual needs.

INTRODUCTION The management of elderly patients is one of the most challenging and ill-considered aspects of health care. Elderly patients with wounds often have a range of other problems which complicate their wound healing and subsequent management as they experience multiple disease processes. In addition, the rate of wound repair generally declines with age, e.g. the inflammatory response, proliferative phase and maturation have all been shown to be delayed (Desai 1997).

Demographic changes are predicted to occur in the UK, with the numbers of elderly people rising rapidly, most growth being in the over-85 age group. Additionally, the number of people aged over 65 years made up 13% of the population in mid-1971 but currently they make up 16% and this figure is expected to increase to 20.5% of the population by the year 2031 (Office for National Statistics 2004).

With the demographic changes forecast for the over-85 age group, elderly people will be the largest group under treatment for most hospital departments (Harding et al 1993). Pressure ulcers developed as a complication of an acute illness episode will therefore become a major concern for all health-care professionals both in hospital and the community (Young & Roper 1996).

Problems associated with increasing age

- Multiple disease processes
- Impaired mobility
- Slower metabolic processes
- Restricted (fixed) incomes
- Lack of medical resources due to finance problems
- Numbers of professional or lay persons available to care for elderly.

PRESSURE ULCERS

Pressure ulcers are a growing problem in an ageing population and can easily arise in the situation described in Case study 8.1.

Case study 8.1

Pressure ulcers

Elsie Mason is an 83-year-old woman who, for the past six years, has been in residential care in a nursing home as her husband found it increasingly difficult to cope. Initially admitted for bouts of forgetfulness and inability to care for herself, her psychological condition has deteriorated dramatically over the last two years and she has recently been diagnosed as having Alzheimer's disease. Whereas previously Elsie had been fairly mobile, she has recently been difficult to mobilize and spends long periods in bed, often missing meals. She has also become incontinent of urine and faeces, failing to indicate to the staff when she wants to go to the toilet. She is often found wandering around at night and is becoming increasingly difficult to communicate with. Her husband is most distressed with her deterioration, especially as she often does not recognize him and tells people he is dead.

Three weeks ago, while Elsie was being bathed, a small red area was noticed on her left hip. Although this was thought insignificant at the time, within four days the whole of the hip had become blackened and lost the outer skin covering. Two weeks later a larger cavity some 12 cm by 10.2 cm and 2 cm deep appeared.

Epidemiology

Up to 20% of elderly patients being nursed in hospital were reported to have pressure ulcers (Norton et al 1975), with this figure rising to 30–66% in orthopaedic and care of the elderly wards (Hibbs 1982, Versluysen 1986). The prevalence in UK hospitals in 1992 was recorded as 6.7% (DoH 1992), rising to 18.6% in 1996 (O'Dea 1995) and falling again to 9.5 % in 1997 (Hanson 1997). So it can be seen that as prevalence rates vary so much, it is difficult to ascertain the real size of the problem. However, there still appears to be a correlation between the **incidence** of pressure ulcers and diseases associated with the ageing process, particularly ischaemic heart disease, peripheral vascular disease and hypertension (Bergstrom & Braden 1992).

Incidence refers to the proportion of a defined group of patients developing pressure ulcers in a defined period of time.

Prevalence refers to the proportion of a defined group of patients with a pressure ulcer in a defined period of time.

Cardiovascular disorders, malnutrition and multiple organ failure adversely affect blood flow, especially to peripheral tissues, which often causes pressure ulcers to develop on the heel (Bliss & Simini 1999). The elderly are particularly vulnerable when undergoing lengthy surgery and require intensive care postoperatively.

Neurological disorders such as Alzheimer's disease and Parkinson's disease can impair mobility and sensation (Bliss 1992). In health the elderly person is highly unlikely to develop a pressure ulcer. It is when an elderly individual becomes ill that they become extremely vulnerable to tissue damage. Such illness is likely to:

- lead to immobility or reduced mobility through spending time in bed, either at home or in hospital
- mean admission to hospital where the patient may be nursed on a hard surface or spend time on X-ray, admission or theatre trolleys
- lead to reduced fluid intake and dehydration
- lead to reduced food intake
- affect the cardiovascular system or neurological system
- produce incontinence.

The above factors predispose the elderly, ill individual to developing pressure ulcers. Even when these factors are transient, tissue damage often has long-term consequences.

The implications for the health and well-being of the elderly patient who develops a pressure ulcer are serious. The cost both to patient and health services in terms of quality of life, morbidity, mortality and resources still remains an enormous problem (EPUAP 1999, NHS 1995).

The cost of managing pressure ulcers is vast and continues to rise. The true cost is unknown but estimated annual costs in the UK were assessed to be around £60 million in 1973, £150 million in 1982 (Scales et al 1982) and £300 million in 1988 (Waterlow 1988). Latest figures from the USA estimate costs of up to $1.3 billion (Gallagher 1997). During the 1990s several documents were produced encouraging a district-wide approach to tackling the problem (Box 8.1). In 1992 *The Health of the Nation* document called for a reduction in pressure ulcers of 5–10% annually (DoH 1992). This prompted many health authorities and trusts to adopt prevention and treatment policies that have in some ways tackled areas of practice that were previously outdated and ineffective (Gebhardt & Bliss 1994). NICE Guideline 7 produced in October 2003 incorporates all available research evidence and previous recommendations in a comprehensive guideline for use by all UK practitioners.

Aetiology   Although pressure ulcers remain a major problem, the exact nature of their development is still poorly understood (NHS 1995).

Many nurses feel sure that they know exactly what constitutes a pressure ulcer but it can be difficult to define the term. Most definitions are broad and do not really address the whole underlying cause. The EPUAP has provided a

Box 8.1 Documents encouraging a district-wide approach to pressure ulcer management

- King's Fund Centre for Health Services Development 1990 The prevention and management of pressure sores within health districts. King's Fund, London
- Department of Health 1992 The Health of the Nation. HMSO, London
- Department of Health 1993 Pressure sores: a key quality indicator. Department of Health, Lancaster
- Touche-Ross & Co, Department of Health 1993 The costs of pressure sores. Department of Health, London
- NHS Centre for Reviews and Dissemination, University of York 1995 The prevention and treatment of pressure sores. Effective Health Care Bulletin 2(1): 1–1
- National Institute for Clinical Excellence 2003 Pressure Ulcer Prevention Clinical Guideline 7. NICE, London

working definition which attempts to give a clearer picture of what a pressure ulcer is: 'A pressure ulcer is an area of localized damage to the skin and underlying tissue caused by pressure, shear, friction and or a combination of these' (EPUAP 1999).

Normal skin

A brief overview of the structure and functions of normal, healthy, undamaged skin follows to help the reader understand the pathogenesis and pathophysiology of pressure ulcer development.

The skin is made up of two layers, the epidermis and the dermis (Figure 8.1). The outer epidermal layer is a barrier, preventing the evaporation of water from the body and absorption of water from the outside environment. The dermal layer also forms a physical barrier preventing the access of bacteria (Powell 1999).

The epidermis consists of dead keratinized cells which are continually being shed from the body and continually replaced from the base of the epidermis. The deeper dermal layer contains blood capillaries, sweat glands, hair follicles and nerve endings. The main functions of the dermis are sensory perception, the control of body temperature and the spread of pressure. The level of anchorage of the epidermis to the dermis varies in thickness and accounts for the greater susceptibility of some parts of the body to the forces of shear and friction. This is called the papillary layer and is thickest on the soles of the feet and palms of the hand.

In healthy individuals, the blood supply to the skin delivers vital oxygen and nutrients and normal sensation is experienced. External pressure occludes the blood vessels, resulting in anoxia. Healthy tissues become devitalized, so causing localized tissue death.

Pressure can be exerted on the tissue in different ways.

- When direct, unrelieved pressure occurs over bony areas. Pressure can be defined as the force exerted perpendicularly over a given area, divided by that

Figure 8.1
Structure of the skin.

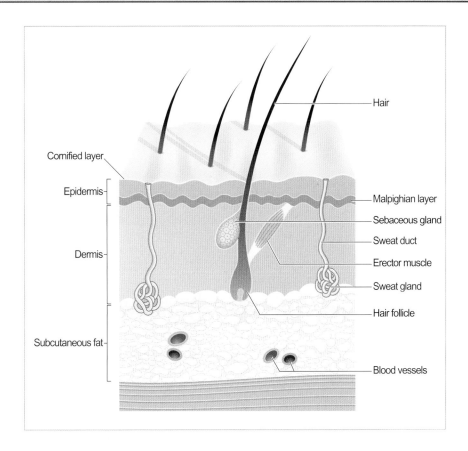

area. Duration of pressure is very important. Tissue damage can occur when high pressure is exerted over an area for a short period or (more often) when lower pressures occur over a prolonged period. The areas covering the bony prominences of the human skeleton are susceptible to such damage owing to there being little tissue to spread the pressure.

■ When friction occurs between the patient's tissues and the hard surface of a bed or chair (Figure 8.2). Typically this can happen when a patient is mishandled and dragged up a bed when being repositioned.

■ When shear force occurs. Shear force is often experienced in combination with friction and direct pressure and happens when tissues are pulled and distorted, disrupting the blood supply to that area. As with pressure, the duration of the shearing is important. Although rigorous shearing can cause tissue necrosis, repeated shearing at a lower level also causes severe tissue damage.

Both shear and friction cause damage to the microcirculation inside the tissue as the dermal and epidermal layers are stretched apart. Extensive damage will result if the lymphatic system has also been damaged as it will be unable to remove the excess amount of interstitial fluid and toxic substances that may have accumulated. This type of damage is not always apparent on the surface skin until some days later. When the epidermal skin finally breaks, to the horror of the carers, a large tortuous cavity may be revealed. The extent of this damage

Figure 8.2
Common sites for pressure ulcer development. (a) Sitting in bed; (b) lying in bed; (c) sitting in a chair.

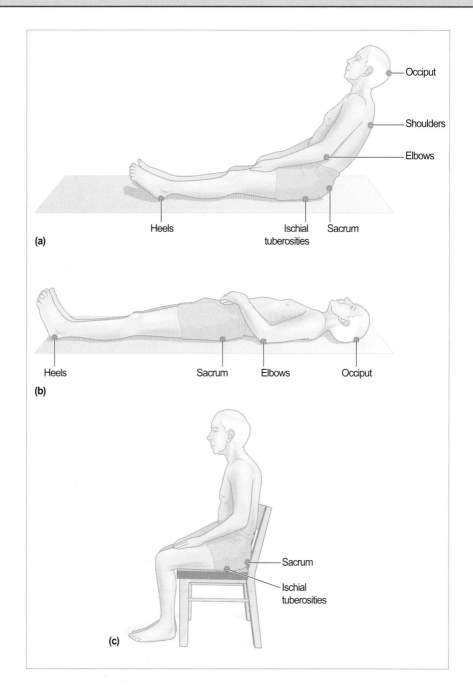

(a)

Occiput

Shoulders

Elbows

Heels

Ischial tuberosities

Sacrum

(b)

Heels

Sacrum

Elbows

Occiput

(c)

Sacrum

Ischial tuberosities

will depend on the length of time the shearing and friction have been allowed to continue unchecked.

Although pressure is the major cause of pressure ulcers, it does not entirely account for the whole pathogenesis of ulcer development (Bliss & Simini 1999).

Other newer theories have recently been suggested, one being that of reactive hyperaemia. This is a normal physiological process that occurs when an area of tissue has been deprived of oxygen. Reperfusion reduces the oxygen

Figure 8.3
Sites of pressure ulcers (figures shown indicate actual number of ulcers counted across countries surveyed) (adapted with kind permission from Clark 2004).

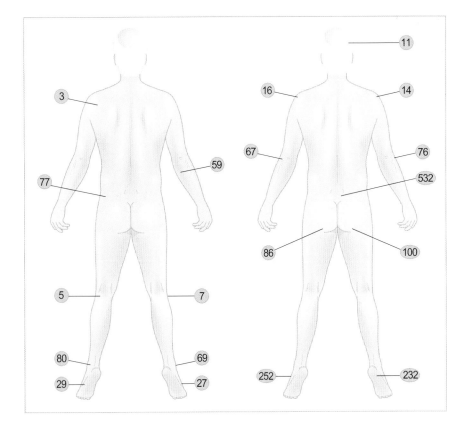

deficiency and removes waste products, thus reducing tissue damage. However, reperfusion to an ischaemic area sees the release of free radicals, toxic substances that are harmful to all kinds of tissue (Bliss 1998). So when an area of the skin has been deprived of oxygen due to pressure, once that pressure is removed, it may be that the sudden inflow of blood to the deprived area causes greater tissue damage due to the release of free radicals than even the pressure itself.

The thinning epidermis of the elderly person also makes the skin very frail; thus mechanical debridement and frequent dressing changes to the pressure ulcers can also cause more damage to the wound and surrounding skin.

A number of research projects have shown the usual location and distribution of pressure ulcers. In the European Pressure Ulcer Advisory Panel's pilot survey within five European countries, the heels and sacrum were the most common sites affected, particularly for Grade 4 (EPUAP classification) (Figure 8.3).

Classification of pressure ulcers

Classification or grading of pressure ulcers is based on the degree of tissue damage observed. Several classifications are available, which has complicated the collection of meaningful data between national and international centres.

The two main classification systems now used have been developed by the American National Pressure Ulcer Advisory Panel (NPUAP 1989) and the European Pressure Ulcer Advisory Panel (EPUAP 1999). The EPUAP was

Figure 8.4
Grade II pressure ulcer.

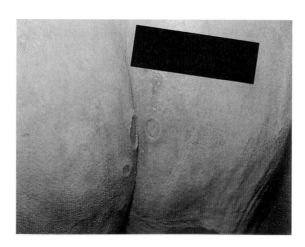

Figure 8.5
Grade III pressure ulcer.

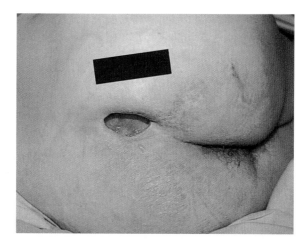

founded in December 1996 and consists of experts from 14 European countries. Since their formation, these bodies have produced prevention and treatment guidelines in which a 1–4 classification of ulcers is presented based on the NPUAP classification. EPUAP has disseminated these guidelines widely and translated them into several languages in the hope that a universal language will be adopted by practitioners throughout Europe.

EPUAP classification
- Grade I: non-blanchable erythema of intact skin. Discolouration of the skin, warmth, oedema, induration or hardness may also be used as indicators, particularly on individuals with darker skin.
- Grade II: partial-thickness skin loss involving epidermis, dermis or both. The ulcer is superficial and presents clinically as an abrasion or blister (Figure 8.4).
- Grade III: full-thickness skin loss involving damage or necrosis of subcutaneous tissue that may extend down to, but not through, underlying fascia (Figure 8.5).

Figure 8.6
Grade IV pressure ulcer.

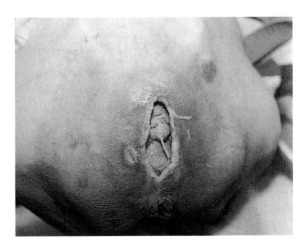

■ Grade IV: extensive destruction, tissue necrosis or damage to muscle, bone or supporting structures with or without full-thickness skin loss (Figure 8.6).

Prevention of pressure ulcers

Most but not all pressure ulcers are preventable (Waterlow 1988). Working on the principle that prevention is better than cure, prevention of pressure ulcers is discussed before treatment and management.

Assessment of risk

Identification of those elderly individuals susceptible to developing pressure ulcers is the first and most important step in preventing tissue breakdown. Clearly, not all elderly people have pressure ulcers so what exactly increases the risk? Important factors are listed in Box 8.2.

Many pressure ulcer risk assessment tools have been devised. Some of these are specifically intended for use with elderly patients, the first and probably the simplest being the Norton scale (Norton et al 1975). Later and more comprehensive scales take into account more factors. One example is the Waterlow scoring system shown in Table 8.1 (Waterlow 1988). This scoring system is available on a washable, plastic card which allows for reuse and easy reassessment.

Box 8.2 What makes older people susceptible to tissue damage?

■ The onset of an intercurrent illness or trauma
■ Immobility, e.g. through illness or orthopaedic surgery
■ Sensory impairment, e.g. diabetes, comatosis, neurological disease
■ Systemic disease, e.g. carcinoma, cardiovascular disease, anaemia
■ Incontinence
■ Dehydration
■ Poor nutrition, malnutrition
■ Patients either below or above average body weight
■ Unrelieved pressure, friction, shearing.

Table 8.1

Waterlow pressure sore prevention/treatment policy card (reproduced with kind permission from Waterlow 1991, revised May 1995)

BUILD/WEIGHT FOR HEIGHT	★	SKIN TYPE VISUAL RISK AREAS	★	SEX AGE	★	SPECIAL RISKS	★
Average	0	Healthy	0	MALE	1	**TISSUE**	★
Above average	1	Tissue paper	1	FEMALE	2	**MALNUTRITION**	
Obese	2	Dry	1	14–49	1	e.g. Terminal cachexia	8
Below average	3	Oedematous	1	50–64	2	Cardiac failure	5
CONTINENCE	★	Clammy (temp ↑)	1	65–74	3	Peripheral vascular	
Complete/	0	Discoloured	2	75–80	4	disease	5
catheterized		Broken/spot	3	81+	5	Anaemia	2
Occasion incontinent	1	**MOBILITY**	★	**APPETITE**	★	Smoking	1
Cath/incontinent	2	Fully mobile	0	Average	0	**NEUROLOGICAL**	★
of faeces		Restless/fidgety	1	Poor	1	**DEFICIT**	
Doubly incontinent	3	Apathetic	2	N.g. tube/	2	e.g. Diabetes, M.S. CVA,	
		Restricted	3	fluids only		Motor/sensory	
		Inert/traction	4	Nbm/anorexic	3	Paraplegia	4–6
		Chairbound	5			**MAJOR SURGERY/ TRAUMA**	★
						Orthopaedic –	5
						Below waist, spinal	
						On table >2 hours	5
						MEDICATION	★
						Cytotoxic drugs	4
						High dose steroids	
						Anti-inflammatory drugs	

SCORE	10+ AT RISK	15+ HIGH RISK	20+ VERY HIGH RISK

RING SCORES IN TABLE, ADD TOTAL. SEVERAL SCORES PER CATEGORY CAN BE USED

N.g. nasogastric

© J Waterlow 1991 Revised May 1995

In 1988 the Braden scale (Braden & Bergstrom 1989), based on the Norton scale, was introduced and today it is probably the most popular scoring system used in the USA (Table 8.2). Risk assessment tools are designed using a combination of risk factors as outlined in Box 8.2 but there is still little known about exactly which are the most important factors. Although Waterlow is used widely in the UK, some practitioners suggest that Braden is a more valid tool for the prediction of ulcer formation (Flanagan 1993).

Nutritional issues in the elderly

In the healthy, elderly individual all tissue is constantly being remodelled or repaired. In the well-nourished individual there is ready availability of proteins, carbohydrates and fats, together with the necessary vitamins and minerals needed for cell metabolism. Poor nutrition interferes with normal metabolic processes, so predisposing the elderly to pressure ulcer formation. When this leads also to weight loss, there is less padding over the bony prominences, so increasing the risk of pressure ulcer development. The nutritional needs of the young and old are identical, apart from energy requirements. The elderly are generally less active and so require less energy (Table 8.3) and also have a reduced basal metabolic rate (Barker 1991).

Table 8.2
The Braden Scale

SENSORY PERCEPTION Ability to respond meaningfully to pressure-related discomfort	1. Completely limited: Unresponsive (doesn't moan, flinch, or gasp) to painful stimuli due to diminished level of consciousness or sedation OR limited ability to feel pain over most of body surface.	2. Very limited: Responds only to painful stimuli. Can't communicate discomfort except by moaning or restlessness OR has a sensory impairment that limits the ability to feel pain or discomfort over half of body.	3. Slightly limited: Responds to verbal commands but can't always communicate discomfort or need to be turned OR has some sensory impairment that limits ability to feel pain or discomfort in one or two extremities.	4. No impairment: Responds to verbal commands. Has no sensory deficit that would limit ability to feel or voice pain or discomfort.
MOISTURE Degree to which skin is exposed to moisture	1. Constantly moist: Skin is kept moist almost constantly by perspiration or urine. Dampness is detected every time patient is moved or turned.	2. Often moist: Skin is often but not always moist. Linen must be changed at least once per shift.	3. Occasionally moist: Skin is occasionally moist, requiring an extra linen change approximately once per day.	4. Rarely moist: Skin is usually dry; linen only requires changing at routine intervals.
ACTIVITY Degree of physical activity	1. Bedfast: Confined to bed.	2. Confined to chair: Ability to walk severely limited or non-existent. Can't bear own weight and must be assisted into chair or wheelchair.	3. Walks occasionally: Walks occasionally during day, but for very short distances, with or without assistance; spends majority of shift in bed or chair.	4. Walks frequently: walks outside the room at least twice per day and inside room at least once every two hours during waking hours.
MOBILITY Ability to change and control body position	1. Completely immobile: Doesn't make even slight changes in body or extremity position without assistance.	2. Very limited: Makes occasional slight changes in body or extremity position but unable to make frequent or significant changes independently.	3. Slightly limited: Makes frequent though slight changes in body or extremity position independently.	4. No limitations: makes major and frequent changes in position without assistance.

Table 8.2
Continued

NUTRITION Usual food intake pattern NPO: Nothing by mouth IV: Intravenously TPN: Total parenteral nutrition	1. Very poor Never eats a complete meal. Rarely eats more than one-third of any food offered. Eats two servings or less of protein (meat or dairy products) per day. Takes fluids poorly. Doesn't take a liquid dietary supplement OR Is NPO or maintained on clear liquids or IV fluids for more than five days.	2. Probably inadequate: Rarely eats a complete meal and generally eats only about half of any food offered. Protein intake includes only three servings of meat or dairy products per day. Occasionally will take a dietary supplement OR receives less than optimum amount of liquid or tube feeding.	3. Adequate: Eats over half of most meals. Eats a total of four servings of protein (meat, dairy product) each day. Occasionally will refuse a meal, but will usually take a supplement if offered OR is on tube feeding or TPN regime that probably meets most nutritional needs.	4. Excellent: eats most of every meal and never refuses a meal. Usually eats a total of four servings of meat and dairy products. Occasionally eats between meals. Doesn't require supplementation.
FRICTION AND SHEAR	1. Problem: Requires moderate to maximum assistance in moving. Complete lifting without sliding against sheet is impossible. Frequently slides down bed or chair, requiring frequent repositioning with maximum assistance. Spasticity, contractures, or agitation leads to almost constant friction.	2. Potential problem: Moves feebly or requires minimum assistance. During a move, skin probably slides to some extent against sheets, chair, restraints, or other devices. Maintains relatively good position in chair or bed most of the time but occasionally slides down.	3. No apparent problem: Moves in bed and chair independently and has sufficient muscle strength to lift up completely during move. Maintains good position in bed or chair at all times.	

Table 8.3
Changes in energy requirements for men and women

Age	Men		Women	
(years)	(kcal)	(kJ)	(kcal)	(kJ)
18	3000	12 600	2200	9240
75+	2100	8 820	1900	7980

The elderly population has been identified as a high-risk group for becoming malnourished (McLaren 1992). Many factors, including lack of motivation, low income and increasing frailty, account for poor-quality food intake. Malnutrition can also be difficult to detect and measure. It is possible that many elderly individuals have some degree of subclinical malnutrition. In a **prevalence** survey carried out by Pinchcofsky-Devin and Kaminski (1986), the overall incidence of malnutrition in the elderly was 59%. This survey also categorized the degree of malnutrition as mild, moderate or severe and found that the elderly patients with pressure ulcers were all in the severely malnourished group.

Apart from the need for appropriate intakes of protein, carbohydrate and fat, some vitamins and minerals are specifically linked with wound healing. It has been suggested that supplements of certain elements increase the rate of tissue repair but there is, as yet, no sound evidence that high doses of any one nutrient will do this (Langer et al 2003). Ascorbic acid (vitamin C) and zinc are two such substances. Vitamin C and zinc deficiency can prevent or delay healing. Patients who are zinc deficient have reduced rates of epithelialization, decreased wound strength and reduced collagen synthesis (Pinchcofsky-Devin 1994). As outlined in Chapter 1, the EPUAP (2003) has recommended certain minimum intakes for patients with wounds, especially pressure ulcers. The blood values of vitamin C and zinc are so difficult to measure that even when deficiencies are suspected, as there is nothing to suggest that supplements of any vitamins or trace elements will aid in healing pressure ulcers, they are best avoided (EPUAP 2004).

When caring for the elderly it may be pertinent to think about the possibility of poor nutrition or malnutrition carefully. With a few simple changes it is possible to improve the diet of an elderly individual (Box 8.3).

PRACTICE POINTS

- Perhaps you have an elderly relative. Find out what their average intake of food is. Look at the whole week. Is the diet balanced and is adequate energy being consumed?
- The next time you are working in this clinical area, select one patient and keep an accurate record of how much and what type of foods the patient is eating.

Incontinence

This is another major factor that increases the risk of pressure ulcer formation in the elderly and measures should be taken to treat incontinence rather than accept it as a consequence of the ageing process.

Box 8.3 Simple changes to improve the diet of the elderly (from Barker 1991)

1. Have a glass of fruit juice every day
2. Have a fortified wholegrain cereal (e.g. Weetabix) with milk for breakfast
3. Try to eat meat or fish once every day
4. Have a milk drink at bedtime
5. Eat at least one serving of vegetables every day

The skin of the incontinent patient is constantly moist which reduces the tissue tolerance of the surface of the skin. This is particularly relevant in the elderly as their skin elasticity is lower and pressure exerted from shear and friction becomes increased within the moist environment.

Skin becomes macerated and excoriated, thus weakening it and making it vulnerable to further damage (Cutting & White 2002).

Equipment for the relief of pressure

A vast array of equipment is available for the relief of pressure, at a wide range of costs. It is therefore understandable that much confusion surrounds this issue. Thankfully, due to the production of the NICE guidelines, many trusts have simplified the management with their own policies outlining exactly which type of equipment should be used for which type of patient.

Equipment tends to fall into two categories.

Low-tech devices These provide a conforming support surface, distributing body weight over a large area. They include:

- standard foam mattress
- alternative foam mattress/overlays
- gel-filled mattress/overlays
- fluid-filled mattress/overlays
- fibre-filled mattress/overlays
- air-filled mattress/overlays.

High-tech devices These are dynamic systems which include:

- alternating-pressure mattress/overlays: patient lies on air-filled sacs which sequentially inflate and deflate, relieving pressure at different anatomical sites for short periods
- air-fluidized beds/mattress/overlays: warmed air is circulated through fine ceramic beads, allowing for support over a large contact area
- low-airloss overlays/mattress/beds: patient is supported on air-filled sacs at constant pressure
- turning beds/frames (kinetic beds): aid manual repositioning or repositioning by motor-driven turning and tilting (Cullum et al 2001).

Considering most pressure ulcers could be prevented, there are still not enough resources allocated to provide the necessary emphasis towards prevention.

ASSESSMENT OF THE ELDERLY PATIENT WITH A PRESSURE ULCER

An elderly individual who has developed a pressure ulcer requires a thorough assessment and rapid nursing intervention. Owing to the nature of the wound, it is inappropriate to deliver a local wound treatment without considering both the physical condition of the elderly individual and the environment in which care is provided. There is a sense of urgency, as the main aim is to prevent further tissue damage while promoting healing. This assessment process precedes the development of a management plan and delivery of care.

Questions to ask

Nutritional status

- Has the patient been receiving adequate nutrition in the past and is the patient currently receiving adequate nutrition? (see above)
- Has the patient's serum **albumin** level been determined? If so, does the level lie within the normal range?
- Does the nutrition of this patient need to be improved?
- Should the dietician be consulted for advice?

Continence

- Is the patient continent of urine and faeces?
- If yes, what can be done to maintain continence?
- If no, how can continence be promoted?
- Should catheterization be considered?
- What types of incontinence aids are available?

Mobility

- What range of mobility does this patient have – full, restricted, limited or none?
- Could mobility be improved with an aid, e.g. Zimmer frame, walking stick, tripod?
- Would physiotherapy help improve mobility?
- What motivation is there to move?

Pressure relief

- What pressure-relieving devices are currently being used to reduce pressure, e.g. foam overlay mattress, chair cushion?
- Is this appropriate for the needs of this patient?
- What is the optimum system for this patient and is it available?
- Does the patient have other areas that are showing signs of pressure?

Wound assessment

A careful examination of the pressure ulcer should be undertaken to determine:

- wound site
- extent of tissue damage
- wound measurement
- health of the wound bed.

Wound site

A chart showing a simple outline of the body can be used to record the site of a pressure ulcer. If more than one ulcer is present, these can be numbered on the chart for more accurate documentation.

The extent of tissue damage

Whatever classification system is used (see above), the grade of pressure ulcer should be assessed and documented directly onto the body chart and/or separately in the nursing notes.

Figure 8.7
Mapping on the skin of a patient with sacral pressure ulcer which shows the undermined area of tissue damage.

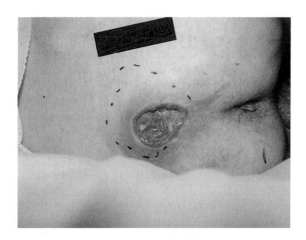

Figure 8.8
Wound measurement: taking a tracing of a pressure ulcer.

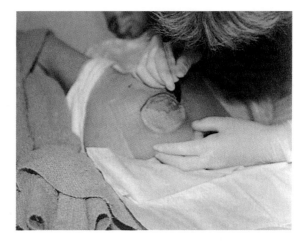

Wound measurement

Measurement of pressure ulcers can be difficult owing to the problems associated with poor wound shape. Tissue damage can spread laterally, undermining the skin (Figure 8.7). The problems associated with undermining include:

- poor exudate drainage predisposing to wound infection and odour
- the possibility of further, devitalized tissue being present which cannot be seen
- difficulties in dressing management.

As accurate an estimation as possible of wound size will help in monitoring the progress or deterioration of the pressure ulcer. Where no undermining or depth occurs, a tracing can be taken (Figure 8.8). Where undermining occurs, the wound opening can be traced, together with the undermined area denoted with a broken line, using forceps to determine the extent of the damage. More frequently now, photographs of the wound site are taken and kept as an accurate record especially when the patient is transferred from one care setting to another.

Figure 8.9
Wound bed with necrotic tissue.

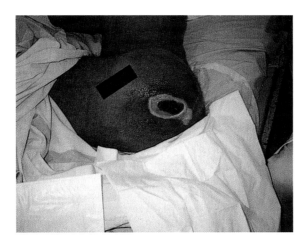

The patient should of course consent to this or their next of kin when informed consent cannot be given.

Health of the wound bed

The appearance of the wound bed is essential in determining the health of the tissues. A range of tissues may be encountered (see Chapter 1).

- Healthy pink or yellow granulation tissue.
- Devitalized tissue, indicating that full wound debridement is not complete.
- Infected tissue. The clinical signs of wound infection are described in Chapter 1. Pressure ulcers are likely to become infected owing to the presence of damaged tissue.
- Dry wound bed: when a pressure ulcer is exposed to the air for long periods, the surface dries out; wound healing can be impaired in the absence of a moist environment.
- Excessively exuding wounds: when large amounts of wound exudate are produced, for example by very extensive pressure ulcers, the skin surrounding the ulcer is susceptible to further tissue damage from becoming macerated.

Meticulous assessment and documentation form the first part of caring for an elderly patient with a pressure ulcer. Further tissue damage should have been eliminated by this stage and management can proceed.

WOUND MANAGEMENT

Having addressed the issues of nutrition, continence, mobility and risk of further tissue damage, the specific management of the pressure ulcer can begin. Although many of the general principles for managing a cavity wound should be taken into account, some additional points require special reference.

- Management of a necrotic pressure ulcer (Figure 8.9). Although this tissue appears to indicate superficial damage, the reverse is often true. Figure 8.10 shows what is happening beneath the surface. Pressure against the bone has caused extensive tissue damage, which has spread laterally. The necrotic area is relatively small and many nurses are surprised that once treatment is initiated the ulcer rapidly extends, revealing an extensive wound (Figure 8.11).

Figure 8.10
Management of a necrotic pressure ulcer. (a) Extent of the damage; (b) necrotic area removed, revealing full extent of the tissue damage; (c) dressing material fills the undermining cavity but is not packed too tightly.

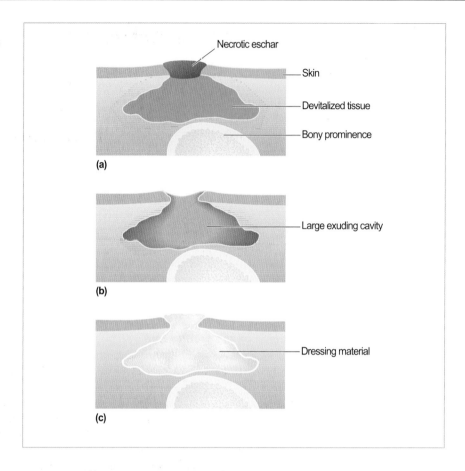

Figure 8.11
The necrotic area is removed, revealing the full extent of tissue damage.

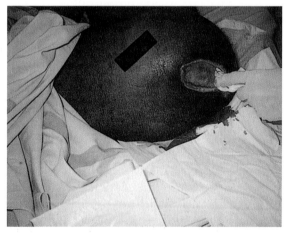

Hydrogel and hydrocolloid materials are useful dressings to effect wound debridement in this type of pressure ulcer. The moistness of these products rehydrates the necrotic area, so facilitating autolysis of the devitalized from the healthy tissue. Over a period of 7–14 days, as the devitalized tissue is removed, the wound may get alarmingly bigger. What is actually

Figure 8.12
Flow chart outlining the management of an older individual with (or at risk of developing) a pressure ulcer.

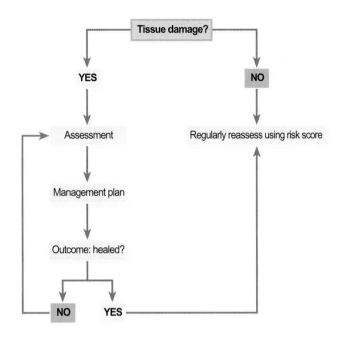

happening is that the devitalized tissue which was already damaged has been removed.

■ Management of undermining (Figure 8.10c). Once the extent of the ulcer has been determined and documented, a material to pack the ulcer under the skin edges is needed. Hard materials such as gauze packing should be avoided as these cause further pressure. Dressing materials such as alginate packing, hydrogel, hydrocolloid pastes, hydrofibre or hydrocellular foam cavity dressings fill the undermining area while creating an environment conducive to healing.

Figure 8.12 shows a flow chart outlining some of the basic steps to take when managing the older individual with, or at risk of developing, a pressure ulcer.

Nursing model for Elsie

It is obvious from Elsie's case study that her interaction with her carers has decreased and that she is often unable to participate actively in her care. When assessing Elsie's problems, the goals should relate to helping her cope with her dependencies in an attempt to achieve some independence.

A number of models could be used for Elsie but probably one of the systems models which stresses the physical side of nursing, such as that of Roper et al (1996), would be best suited to a patient like Elsie. Although each part is studied separately, the interaction between these parts is most important.

As always, the nurse must set priorities of care when using the 12 assessment areas. Although the wound may seem the most important area, the potential for healing will be impaired if Elsie's nutritional status is ignored. Remember, too, that Elsie is being cared for in a nursing home, where levels of trained staff may be low. Care should be straightforward and manageable for all involved.

Table 8.4
Assessment of Elsie's usual routine (Case study 8.1)

Activity of living	Problem statement
Maintaining a safe environment	Often wanders around at night
Communicating	Slightly deaf, wears glasses Does not communicate clearly, often talks to herself, does not recognize people
Breathing	Breathes easily, no chest problems Blood pressure within normal limits
Eating and drinking	Malnourished Needs to be reminded and encouraged to eat and drink Lacks interest in food – 'plays' with it
Eliminating	Incontinent of urine during day and night Occasionally incontinent of faeces at night
Personal cleansing and dressing	Will sometimes wash herself Often dresses without regard to items Skin often excoriated with urine
Controlling body temperature	Normal temperature
Mobilizing	Spends long periods of time in bed Has pressure ulcer on right hip
Working and playing	Sometimes joins in with home's activities but often sits by herself
Expressing sexuality	Does not always recognize husband, thinks he is dead on occasions
Sleeping	Often awake during the night, sleeps during the day
Dying	Expresses wish to die on occasions

The assessment of Elsie's activities of living is given in Table 8.4 and the care plan in Table 8.5.

PRACTICE POINTS

- It is important to note that, although the care for Elsie was comprehensive, she is at constant risk of developing further ulcers, as are many of the other residents in the home.
- Education is an important factor for the staff of the home and community nursing input should aim to provide a programme of support and advice to the matron and staff.

Table 8.5
Care plan based on problems identified in Table 8.4

Activity of living	Problem	Goal	Intervention
Mobilizing	Pressure ulcer cavity 6 cm × 2 cm containing necrotic tissue (A)	Promote healing with removal of necrotic tissue	Debride wound with combined use of hydrogel and surgical debridement
	Infection in cavity (P)	Eliminate infection	1. Take would swab 2. Doctor to prescribe appropriate antibiotics 3. Apply principles of asepsis; avoid cross-contamination
	Lacks motivation to mobilize (A) Further skin breakdown (P)	Prevent shear forces and direct pressure 1. Keep skin clean 2. Promote wound healing 3. Eliminate extrinsic factors	Involve Elsie in home's activities. Encourage mixing with other residents 1. Assess with Risk Assessment Tool 2. Instal appropriate pressure-relieving equipment 3. Change position and mobilize 2-hourly during day, change position 4-hourly at nights. Daily shower or bath. Ensure all staff familiar with regiment
Eating and drinking	Malnourished (A) Further protein breakdown (P)	1. Counteract effects of catabolism 2. Promote wound healing	1. Refer to community dietician for assessment 2. Give 3000–4000 kcal (12600–16800 kJ) with high-protein supplement 3. Staff to monitor mealtimes
Eliminating	Incontinent of urine and faeces (A) Skin maceration increasing risk of friction (P)	1. Restore continence 2. Prevent further skin breakdown	1. Staff to toilet Elsie every 2 hours 2. Rule out urinary tract infection or faecal retention 3. Avoid drinks before bedtime, toilet before bedtime 4. Wash skin thoroughly if contaminated 5. Avoid use of incontinence sheets or pads
Communicating	Difficulty in communicating needs	Maintain level of reality orientation	1. Speak clearly and always talk in the present 2. Avoid use of reminiscence 3. Inform Elsie of all nursing actions, involving her husband in care where possible 4. Ensure husband understands the nature of the disease process
Sleeping	Disturbed sleep pattern (A)	Restore normal pattern of 6 hours per night	1. Keep Elsie active in the daytime 2. Do not allow her to sleep during the day 3. Establish a bedtime routine
Expressing sexuality	Husband separated from wife – feels guilty at leaving her in a nursing home	Restore role for husband	Give husband tasks to aid his wife's recovery, e.g. feeding at mealtimes, and toileting during the day

(A), actual problem; (P), potential problem.

SUMMARY

There is much to think about in order that patients are managed with the optimum level of care. Management requires the skill and expertise of many health team members, whether the patient is in hospital or the community. It is important that you become a team member and learn when to use the other team members' expertise, as follows:

- Dietician: ensures type and level of protein and carbohydrates appropriate to patient's needs.
- Occupational therapist: supplies pressure-relieving equipment.
- Physiotherapist: ensures muscle wasting and contractures are kept to a minimum.
- Tissue viability nurse: available for specialist advice and may be responsible for protocol development.
- Plastic surgeon: required for healing of pressure ulcers.
- Physician, surgeon: controls intrinsic factors such as diabetes, urinary incontinence.
- Generalist nurse: coordinates plan of care; educates patient and relatives.

A planned programme of care will include all these people. Recognition of predisposing factors and early signs of pressure ulcer development outlined in this chapter will contribute to the lowering of the incidence and prevalence of pressure ulcers.

Could *you* recognize them?

FURTHER READING

Baranoski S, Ayello E A 2004 Wound care essentials: practice principles. Lippincott, Williams and Wilkins, Springhouse, Pennsylvania.

Barton A, Barton M 1978 The management and prevention of pressure sores. Faber and Faber, London.

Clark M (ed) 2004 Pressure ulcers: recent advances in tissue viability. Quay Books, Salisbury.

Phillips J 1997 Access to clinical education: pressure sores. Churchill Livingstone, Edinburgh.

Versluysen M 1986 How elderly patients with femoral neck fractures develop pressure sores in hospital. British Medical Journal 292: 1311–1313.

REFERENCES

Barker H M 1991 Nutrition and the elderly. Beck's nutrition and dietetics for nurses. Churchill Livingstone, Edinburgh.

Bergstrom N, Braden B 1992 A prospective study of pressure sore risk amongst institutional elderly. Journal of the American Geriatric Society 40: 747–758.

Bliss M 1992 Acute pressure area care: Sir Thomas Paget's legacy. Lancet 339: 221–223.

Bliss M 1998 Hyperaemia. Journal of Tissue Viability 8(4): 4–13.

Bliss M, Simini B 1999 When are the seeds of postperative pressure sores sown? British Medical Journal 319: 863–864.

Braden B, Bergstrom N 1989 Clinical utility of the Braden Scale for predicting pressure sore risk. Decubitus 2(3): 44–51.

Clark M (ed) 2004 Pressure ulcers: recent advances in tissue viability. Quay Books, Salisbury.

Cullum N, Nelson E A, Sheldon T 2001 Systematic reviews of wound care (5): pressure-relieving beds, mattresses and cushions for the prevention and treatment of pressure sores. Health Technology Assessment 5:9.

Cutting K F, White R J 2002 Maceration of the skin: 1: the nature and causes of skin maceration. Journal of Wound Care 11(7): 275–278.

Desai H 1997 Ageing and wounds part 2: healing in old age. Journal of Wound Care 6(5): 237–239.

Department of Health 1992 The Health of the Nation. HMSO, London.

European Pressure Ulcer Advisory Panel (EPUAP) 1999 Pressure ulcer prevention guidelines. EPUAP, Oxford.

European Pressure Ulcer Advisory Panel (EPUAP) 2003 EPUAP guidelines on the role of nutrition in pressure ulcer prevention and management. EPUAP Review 5(2): 50–53.

European Pressure Ulcer Advisory Panel (EPUAP) 2004 Pressure ulcers and nutrition: a new European guideline. Journal of Wound Care 13(7): 267–272.

Flanagan M 1993 Predicting pressure sore risk. Journal of Wound Care 2(4): 215–218.

Gallagher S 1997 Outcomes in clinical practice: pressure ulcer prevalence and incidence studies. Ostomy and Wound Management 43: 28–38.

Gebhardt K S, Bliss M R 1994 Preventing pressure sores in orthopaedic patients. Is prolonged chain nursing detrimental? Journal of Tissue Viability 4: 51–54.

Hanson R 1997 Sore points sorted. Nursing Times 92 (7): 66–72.

Harding K G, Jones V, Sinclair A J 1993 Wound care in an ageing population. Journal of Wound Care 2(6): 346.

Hibbs P 1982 Pressure sores: a system of prevention. Nursing Mirror 155(5): 25–29.

Langer G, Schloemer G, Knerr A et al 2003 Nutritional interventions for preventing and treating pressure ulcers. The Cochrane Library, Issue 4. Update Software, Oxford.

McLaren S M G 1992 Nutrition and wound healing. Journal of Wound Care 1(3): 45–55.

National Pressure Ulcer Advisory Panel (NPUAP) 1989 Pressure ulcers: prevalence, cost and risk assessment. Consensus Development Conference statement. Decubitus 2: 24–35.

NHS Centre for Reviews and Dissemination, University of York 1995 The prevention and treatment of pressure sores. Effective Health Care Bulletin 21: 1–16.

Norton D, McLaren R, Exton-Smith A N 1975 An investigation of geriatric nursing problems in hospital. Churchill Livingstone, Edinburgh.

O'Dea K 1995 The prevalence of pressure sores in four European countries. Journal of Wound Care 4 (4): 192–195.

Office for National Statistics 2004 National statistics. Available online at: www.statistics.gov.uk.

Pinchcofsky-Devin G 1994 Nutritional wound healing. Journal of Wound Care 3(5): 231–234.

Pinchcofsky-Devin G, Kaminski M V 1986 Correlation of pressure sores and nutritional status. Journal of the American Geriatric Society 34: 435–440.

Powell J 1999 Physiology of the skin. Surgery 17(3): IV-VII.

Roper N, Logan W, Tierney A 1996 The elements of nursing, 4th edn. Churchill Livingstone, Edinburgh.

Scales J T, Lowthian P J, Poole A G 1982 'Vaperm' patient support system: a new general purpose hospital mattress. Lancet 2: 1150–1152.

Versluysen M 1986 How elderly patients with femoral neck fractures develop pressure sores in hospital. British Medical Journal 292: 1311–1313.

Waterlow J 1988 Prevention is cheaper than cure. Nursing Times 84(25): 69–70.

Young J, Roper T A 1996 The role of the doctor in the management of pressure sores. Journal of Tissue Viability 7(1): 18–19.

Wound care in the elderly individual with leg ulceration and malignancy

KEY ISSUES This chapter looks at wounds other than pressure ulcers that are common in the elderly population.

Clinical Case Studies
Aetiology and management of:

■ an independent woman suffering with venous ulceration
■ the onset of arterial ulceration in an elderly man
■ advanced stages of breast disease in a lady with a fungating breast tumour.

PRACTICE POINTS As you read through this chapter, concentrate on the following:

■ the importance of the nurse–patient relationship in helping patients understand the nature of their wounds
■ the importance of correct assessment when dealing with patients with leg ulceration
■ palliative management of a wound when healing is not the outcome
■ the importance of understanding the basic principles of wound management.

INTRODUCTION The general problems of wound management in the elderly patient were discussed in the introduction to Chapter 8. This chapter concentrates on the problems of leg ulceration and malignancy.

LEG ULCERATION It has been estimated that in 1992 around 400 000 patients in the UK had experienced leg ulceration, 100 000 of whom currently required treatment (Fletcher 1992). Leg ulceration affects about 0.15% of the population in the UK (Callam et al 1985) and the prevalence increases with age, from 10 per 1000 within the adult population to 36 per 1000 in the over-65 age group, particularly in women (Table 9.1).

The estimated costs of treating leg ulcer patients range from £230 million to £400 million per annum in the UK (Bosanquet 1992). A high proportion of these costs is spent on dressings and district nurse time, with district nurses

Figure 9.1
Aetiology of leg ulcers.

Table 9.1
Increasing prevalence of leg ulcers in women with advancing age (reproduced with kind permission from Callam 1999)

Age (years)	Male–female ratio
Under 65	1 : 1
65–74	1 : 2.6
75–84	1 : 4.8
85+	1 : 10.3

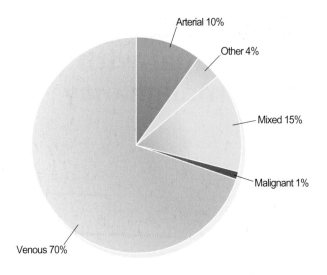

Arterial 10%

Other 4%

Mixed 15%

Malignant 1%

Venous 70%

spending 10–50% of their time managing leg ulcer patients (Morison & Moffatt 1994). Only 1% of leg ulcer patients are managed in hospital (Callam et al 1985). The implications of this are that patients with leg ulceration are treated in the community, with district nurses providing day-to-day care for these patients and also acting as a facilitator for other services (Callam 1999).

The aetiology of leg ulcers is shown in Figure 9.1. One percent of these ulcers may be malignant (Figure 9.2).

VENOUS ULCERS

In the elderly population, venous disease is the major cause of leg ulceration. A case of venous ulceration is described in Case study 9.1.

Case study 9.1

Venous ulcers

Joan Knight, an independent 73-year-old retired headteacher, is an active member of the village community in which she has lived and taught all her life. Although now widowed and living alone, she has much social contact. While helping to serve tea at the local summer fête she scraped her leg on the tea trolley. The laceration bled profusely but having enlisted the aid of a friend to stop the bleeding, Joan thought no more about it. She treated the wound herself with an old remedy of cold tea soaks and a bandage but, six weeks later, was dismayed to find that the wound had developed into a deep crater which was producing lots of exudate and smelt rather unpleasant.

She reluctantly went to her general practitioner who seemed to be more interested in asking her about when she had had her children than the wound itself. Joan recalled that after the birth of both children she had a condition called 'white leg'.

The doctor sent her to the district nurse's room, where blood was taken, the wound measured and the ankle brachial pressure index in the affected leg was recorded.

Figure 9.2
A malignant ulcer.

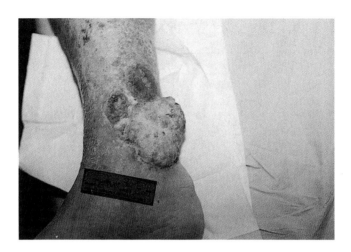

Aetiology

In health the venous system of the lower leg pumps blood back towards the heart. As this action takes place against gravity in the human, this is difficult to achieve.

There are three categories of vein within the legs: deep, superficial and communicating (perforator) veins. The superficial long and short saphenous veins (draining the skin) pump blood under low pressure into the deep venous system through the perforators (Figure 9.3). The deep veins are surrounded by muscles (the calf muscle pump) which contract and relax during walking to pump blood up the leg. Healthy venous return is achieved not only by walking (so using the calf muscle pump) but also by having full ankle movement; when the ankle moves, the Achilles tendon contracts and releases, to assist the calf muscle pump.

Damage to the venous system can occur at any time of life. Deep vein thrombosis and varicose veins damage the perforators, making them incompetent (Figure 9.4). Immobility of and arthritic changes to the ankle joint impair ankle movement and so further impede venous return.

Failure of the calf muscle pump results in backflow of blood and pooling, causing venous hypertension, which leads to oedema of the lower leg and pigmentation of the 'gaiter' area (Cullum 1994). This pigmentation is the result of haemoglobin being released from red blood cells which have leaked out of the distended blood capillaries and deposited haemosiderin. Also, the subsequent rise in ambulatory pressure is believed to enlarge and increase the permeability of the local capillary bed, allowing molecules such as fibrinogen to escape into the interstitial fluid. Fibrinogen is then formed into insoluble fibrin complexes which forms a cuff around capillaries, affecting oxygen diffusion into the tissues. This so-called 'fibrin cuff theory' was first proposed by Burnand et al (1976). The gradual replacement of skin and subcutaneous tissue by fibrous tissue also explains the appearance of 'woody skin', a condition called lipodermatosclerosis so commonly seen in patients with venous ulceration (Browse 1983).

Other explanations for causation have been given, mostly related to the 'white cell trapping' theory (Coleridge-Smith et al 1988), where it is believed that following an episode of deep vein thrombosis or phlebitis, white cells

Figure 9.3
The normal venous
system of the leg.

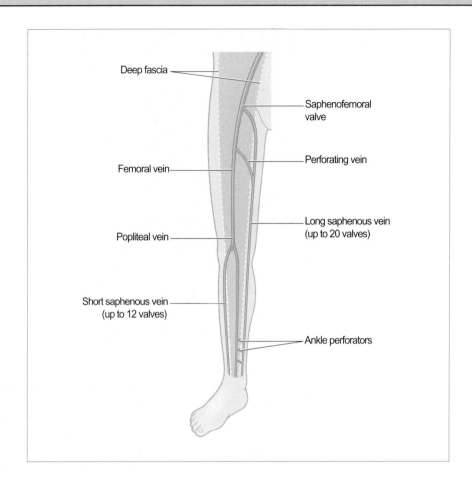

Deep fascia

Saphenofemoral
valve

Perforating vein

Femoral vein

Long saphenous vein
(up to 20 valves)

Popliteal vein

Short saphenous vein
(up to 12 valves)

Ankle perforators

Figure 9.4
A damaged venous
system: an incompetent
valve in a perforating vein
allows backflow of blood
from the deep to the
superficial venous system.

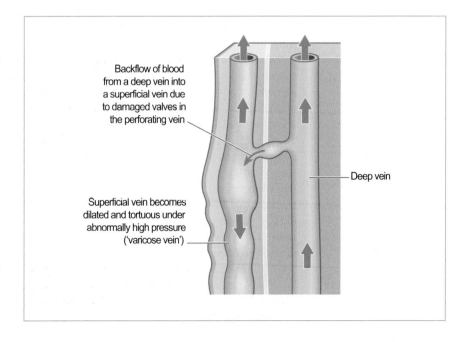

Backflow of blood
from a deep vein into
a superficial vein due
to damaged valves in
the perforating vein

Deep vein

Superficial vein becomes
dilated and tortuous under
abnormally high pressure
('varicose vein')

Figure 9.5
A venous leg ulcer showing ulceration of the gaiter area.

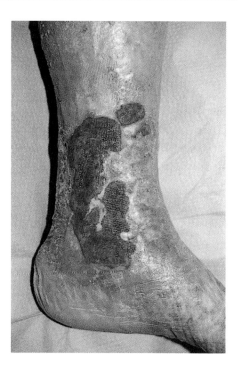

increase and become trapped in the capillaries of the leg. Here they release toxic substances such as oxygen free radicals, causing tissue death. This underlying problem is soon revealed as any subsequent knock or minor injury to this area of the lower leg can rapidly lead to ulceration. Ulceration most commonly occurs around the gaiter area (Figure 9.5) where usually the ulcers are shallow. A medical history of damage to the venous system may typically include previous phlebitis, deep vein thrombosis, severe leg injury, including a fracture, or varicose veins. These ulcers may take months to heal and patients are susceptible to recurrence at a later date .

Assessment of an ulcerated limb

The aim of assessment is to exclude other causes of leg ulceration and to confirm a diagnosis of venous ulceration. Effective management depends on an accurate diagnosis. As only 1% of patients with leg ulceration are managed in hospital, this assessment takes place either in the community or in an outpatient department (Callam et al 1985).

History taking, examination and investigations form this assessment and ideally are undertaken by a multidisciplinary team.

History taking

A comprehensive medical history is taken specifically to detect venous disease and exclude other causes of ulceration (Table 9.2).

Examination

A physical examination is undertaken to support the medical history and to identify possible health problems which have gone unrecognized. Both legs should be examined, not just the ulcerated limb. Examination will include the following points.

Table 9.2
The patient's history may indicate the cause of ulceration

Indicates venous disease	Indicates other cause of ulceration

History of:
   deep vein thrombosis
   pulmonary embolism
   previous vein surgery
   fractures of the leg
	History of:
	   diabetes (mellitus)
	   vascular surgery and/or disease
	   intermittent claudication
	   rest pain

Year of first ulcer	
Number of previous episodes of ulceration	
Time this ulcer has been present	

Table 9.3
Investigations of leg ulceration

Investigations often undertaken	Possible further investigations
Palpation of pedal or posterior tibial pulses	Blood profiles, e.g. blood glucose level, full blood count, U & E, LFT, rheumatoid factor
Brachial blood pressure and leg systolic pressure, ankle brachial pressure index	Duplex scan
Measurement of the ulcer by tracing or photography	Venography
Measurement of ankle and leg circumference	Wound swab if infection suspected
Documentation of the ulcer site, wound bed, exudate level, previous dressings used, compression bandages used	Patch testing to determine if patient has allergies

- Is the shape of the leg normal or 'champagne bottle' shaped, oedematous or thin?
- Is the surrounding skin normal, smooth and well hydrated or eczematous, scratched, pigmented by haemosiderin, lipodermatosclerosis or with varicose veins?
- Is the ankle joint fully mobile, of limited mobility or completely fixed?

Investigations

The investigations listed in Table 9.3 form part of the assessment process and should not be used as the only method of determining a diagnosis.

Doppler ultrasonographic assessment

1. Make the patient comfortable. The patient should be lying flat (if possible for 15–20 minutes before the procedure).
2. Locate the brachial pulse with the **Doppler ultrasonograph**, apply ultrasound gel and inflate the sphygmomanometer cuff. When the signal fades and disappears, gradually deflate the cuff and record the point at which the signal returns (brachial systolic pressure).
3. Examine the dorsal area of the ulcerated limb and locate the dorsalis pedis pulse (note that this is absent in around 12% of the population). If no pedal pulse can be located, use the posterior tibial pulse. Apply the sphygmomanometer cuff just above the ankle, warning the patient that this procedure

Figure 9.6
Using a hand-held
Doppler probe.

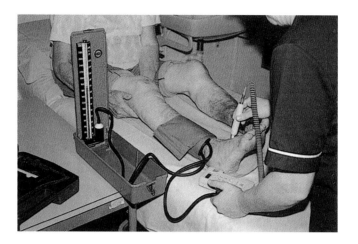

may be uncomfortable for a few minutes. Apply ultrasound gel and inflate the cuff, listening carefully for the signal to disappear. Again, gradually deflate the cuff, noting and recording the point at which the signal returns (ankle systolic pressure) (Figure 9.6).

$$\frac{\text{ankle systolic pressure}}{\text{brachial systolic pressure}} = \text{ankle brachial pressure index}$$

A reasonable guide to using Doppler assessment (in conjunction with a full physical examination and history taking) is to use the ankle brachial pressure index (APBI) to confirm your clinical opinion (Figure 9.7). If the ABPI is considered to confirm the diagnosis, then a patient with an index of 0.8 or more will benefit from the use of compression therapy, whereas an ABPI below 0.8 is not generally considered suitable for compression (RCN 1998).

Management

The principles of managing patients with venous ulceration lie in controlling or compensating for the damaged venous system. Although the ulcer will require a dressing, the bandaging system and compression therapy are by far the most important aspect of care. Supporting the damaged venous system using graduated compression aims to provide greater support at the ankle and less towards the knee and is the most effective method of compensating for damaged veins (NHS 1997).

For patients with venous ulceration, dressing materials play a far less important role than the compression bandages. Patients do find this a difficult concept to understand, focusing on the wound itself rather than the underlying pathology in the limb. Depending on assessment of the wound, any of the modern wound dressing materials may be suitable as a primary wound contact layer. The low-adherent dressings, either non-medicated or medicated, hydrophilic foams and alginates are popular, as these products can be left in place for several days at a time (Figures 9.8–9.11).

Bandages cause two different types of pressure on the leg:

■ resting: pressure extended when leg is at rest
■ ambulatory: pressure exerted during muscle work.

Dopplex Ankle Pressure Index (API) Guide

Ankle Pressure (mmHg)

Brachial Pressure (mmHg)	30	35	40	45	50	55	60	65	70	75	80	85	90	95	100	105	110	115	120	125	130	135	140	145	150	155	160	165	170	175	180	185	190	195	200	
180	.16	.19	.22	.25	.27	.30	.33	.36	.38	.41	.44	.47	.50	.52	.55	.58	.61	.63	.66	.69	.72	.75	.77	.80	.83	.86	.89	.92	.94	.97	1.00					180
175	.17	.20	.22	.25	.28	.31	.34	.37	.40	.42	.45	.48	.51	.54	.57	.60	.62	.65	.68	.71	.74	.77	.80	.82	.85	.88	.92	.94	.97	1.00						175
170	.17	.20	.23	.26	.29	.32	.35	.38	.41	.44	.47	.50	.52	.55	.58	.61	.64	.67	.70	.73	.76	.79	.82	.85	.89	.91	.94	.97	1.00							170
165	.18	.21	.24	.27	.30	.33	.36	.39	.42	.45	.48	.51	.54	.57	.60	.63	.66	.69	.72	.75	.78	.81	.84	.87	.90	.94	.96	1.00								165
160	.18	.21	.25	.28	.31	.34	.37	.40	.43	.46	.50	.53	.56	.59	.62	.65	.68	.71	.75	.78	.81	.84	.87	.90	.93	.96	1.00									160
155	.19	.22	.25	.29	.32	.35	.38	.41	.45	.48	.51	.54	.58	.61	.64	.67	.70	.74	.76	.80	.83	.87	.90	.93	.96	1.00										155
150	.20	.23	.26	.30	.33	.36	.40	.43	.46	.50	.53	.56	.60	.63	.66	.70	.73	.76	.80	.83	.86	.90	.93	.96	1.00											150
145	.20	.24	.27	.31	.34	.37	.41	.44	.48	.51	.55	.58	.62	.65	.69	.72	.75	.79	.82	.86	.90	.93	.96	1.00												145
140	.21	.25	.28	.32	.35	.39	.42	.46	.50	.53	.57	.60	.64	.67	.71	.75	.78	.82	.85	.89	.92	.96	1.00													140
135	.22	.26	.29	.33	.37	.40	.44	.48	.51	.55	.59	.62	.66	.70	.74	.77	.81	.85	.88	.92	.96	1.00														135
130	.23	.27	.30	.34	.38	.42	.46	.50	.53	.57	.61	.65	.69	.73	.77	.80	.84	.88	.92	.96	1.00															130
125	.24	.28	.32	.36	.40	.44	.48	.52	.56	.60	.64	.68	.72	.76	.80	.84	.88	.92	.96	1.00																125
120	.25	.29	.33	.37	.40	.45	.50	.54	.58	.62	.66	.70	.75	.79	.83	.87	.91	.95	1.00																	120
115	.26	.30	.34	.39	.43	.48	.52	.56	.60	.65	.69	.74	.78	.82	.86	.91	.95	1.00																		115
110	.27	.31	.36	.40	.45	.50	.54	.59	.63	.68	.72	.77	.81	.86	.90	.95	1.00																			110
105	.28	.33	.38	.42	.47	.52	.57	.61	.66	.71	.76	.80	.85	.90	.95	1.00																				105
100	.30	.35	.40	.45	.50	.55	.60	.65	.70	.75	.80	.85	.90	.95	1.00																					100

GREATER THAN 1.00

HNE Diagnostics, a world leading manufacturer of pocket Dopplers, offers an extensive range of bi-directional pocket Dopplers with visual flow and rate display, together with a wide range of interchangeable probes for both vascular and obstetric applications.

WARNING: False high readings may be obtained in patients with calcified arteries because the sphygmomanometer cuff cannot fully compress the hardened arteries. Calcified arteries may be present in patients with history of Diabetes, Arteriosclerosis and Atherosclerosis.

$$API = \frac{\text{Ankle systolic pressure}}{\text{Brachial systolic pressure}}$$

Note: Diastolic pressure cannot be measured using a Doppler.

HNE DIAGNOSTICS

Recommended Probe Frequencies:
8 MHz for normal sized limbs
5 MHz for obese / oedematous limbs

35 Portmanmoor Road, Cardiff, CF2 2HB, UK. Tel: +44 (0)1222 485885 Fax: +44 (0)1222 492520
® Dopplex, Flowtron and 'H' logo are registered trademarks of Huntleigh Technology plc in the UK, and in some cases, other territories.

A member of the Huntleigh Technology plc Group of companies. © Copyright Huntleigh Technology plc 1995

6AH239-1

Figure 9.7
Ankle pressure index guide (reproduced with kind permission of Huntleigh Healthcare, Cardiff).

Figure 9.8
Tissue necrosis caused by a compression bandage applied to a leg with a poor blood supply.

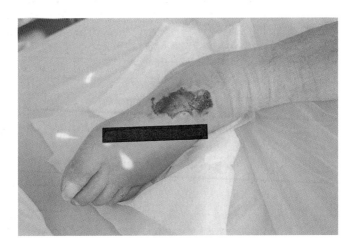

Figure 9.9
A venous leg ulcer treated with a paste bandage.

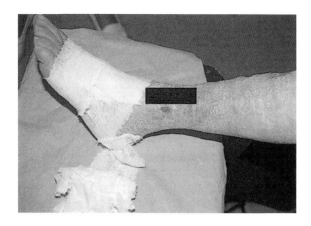

Figure 9.10
Multilayer bandaging system (Charing Cross four-layer).

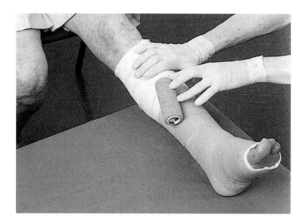

Compression bandages fall into two categories.

- Elastic (long stretch): these contain an elastomer, allowing the fibres to stretch with movement without losing pressure.
- Inelastic (short stretch): these contain no elastomeric fibres and depend on crimped threads for their extensibility. These exert higher pressures when the patient is walking but much less when they are at rest (Finnie 2002).

These bandages are further grouped depending on the level of compression they exert which can vary from 14 to 50 mmHg. See Table 9.4 on type 3 compression bandage types.

They should only be applied following an in-depth assessment and by experienced and trained practitioners. Inadequate bandage technique may not achieve the right level of compression and can have serious implications (Finnie 2002) (see Figure 9.8).

Graduated compression hosiery has an important role in following the treatment of a venous leg ulcer and should also be encouraged to prevent recurrence (NHS 1997).

Compression stockings are fitted following measurement of the limb. It is imperative that the patient is measured correctly and therefore it is usual for

Figure 9.11
Applying compression bandages in a figure of eight. (a) Maintain foot at a right angle to the leg. (b) Make two turns at the base of the toes. (c) Take bandage above the heel. (d) Take bandage around the heel to cover the foot. (e, f) Continue bandaging using figure-of-eight turns. Ensure that 50% stretch is maintained. (g) Bandage up to the tibial tuberosity.

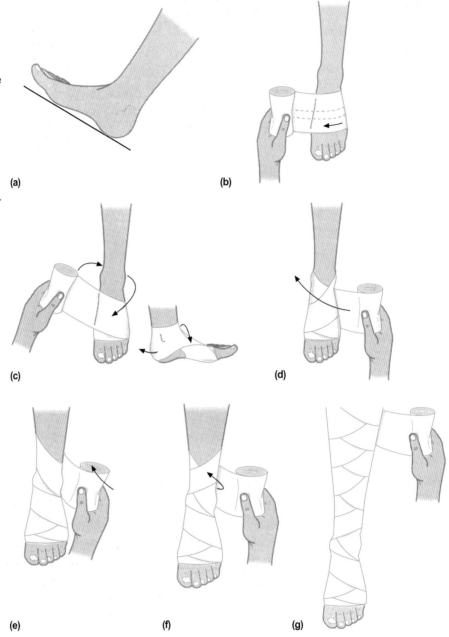

(a)

(b)

(c)

(d)

(e)

(f)

(g)

the appliance department or a trained community pharmacist to fit patients with compression stockings.

Physiotherapy

Physiotherapy may be indicated for patients who have limited mobility, limited ankle movement or fixed joints. More mobile patients should be encouraged to walk and exercise as much as possible (Figures 9.12–9.14). Prolonged standing should be avoided at all costs as this further impedes venous return.

Table 9.4
Type 3 compression bandages (adapted from Finnie 2002)

Type 3a	Light compression 14–17 mmHg at the ankle	Good for early varicose veins, not suitable for reducing oedema or for large limbs
Type 3b	Moderate compression 18–24 mmHg at the ankle	Treatment and prevention of ulcers and control of mild oedema
Type 3c	High compression 25–35 mmHg at the ankle	Maintains high levels of compression in patients who have bigger legs and are active

Figure 9.12
Exercises for assisting venous return: marking time while standing still.

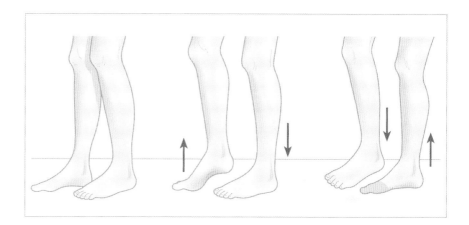

Motivation and patient education

Recurrence rates for venous ulcers can be almost as high as 100% (Mayberry et al 1991). This high rate is in part due to the lack of patient compliance with their treatment (Moffatt 2004).

The key to success in managing patients with venous ulceration lies in involving the patient with their treatment. The nurse will provide dressings and compression but it is the patient who is responsible for exercise and tolerance of the compression system. Patients can best help themselves if they receive appropriate information and advice and are truly integrated into their care. Although many patients will be treated in their own home by the district nurse, some patients can attend one of the many leg ulcer clinics that are now available throughout the UK. The first clinic to offer specialist management was established by Christine Moffatt in 1989. This clinic crossed the boundaries of community care and patient assessment with access to vascular services at Charing Cross Hospital. Many have followed this model but further developments have been made by Ellie Lindsay who has established the concept of Leg Clubs® as a way of empowering patients to take ownership of their treatment (Lindsay 2001). The ethos of such groups is that the patient is the central focus and as such directs their own management.

Figure 9.13
Exercises for assisting venous return: walking as much as possible.

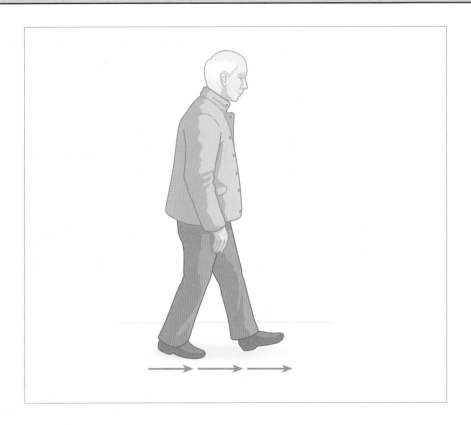

Figure 9.14
Exercises for assisting venous return: rotate ankles in a circular motion, first one way and then the other.

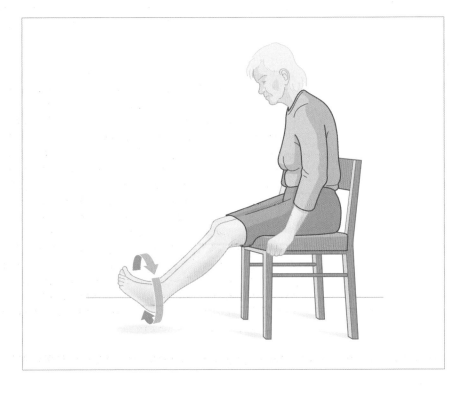

Nursing model for Joan

When choosing a model of care for an individual such as Joan, it is important to consider the type of person the nurse is caring for. As the case study indicates, Joan is an intelligent, independent lady. She is used to telling people what to do and 'doing' for herself. Joan needs a model that focuses on the *interaction* between nurse and patient. One that focuses on the patient's perception of the situation would be Riehl's interaction model (Riehl 1980). This model also addresses the person's interaction with their environment. Joan now has to adapt and change the way she interacts, as her normal pattern of behaviour has undergone a change. Using this model, attempt to assess Joan's problems and design a plan of care to meet her needs.

PRACTICE POINTS

- Joan's mainstay of treatment is compression therapy. This requires both patient understanding of the treatment and compliance.
- This should not present a problem in Joan's case as long as she is treated as a true partner in care.

ARTERIAL ULCERS

Although not as common as venous ulceration, the arterial ulcer (Case study 9.2) is considerably more problematic for patients.

Case study 9.2

Arterial ulcers

Mr Jack Jones is an 83-year-old man who worked down the mines from the age of 15 years until he was 60 years old. A smoker all his life, his physical condition is poor, with frequent bouts of bronchitis during the winter due to pneumoconiosis. He lives with his wife in a small terraced house and his only social outing is a weekly visit to the servicemen's club for a game of darts.

Although the club is only at the end of the street, Jack has found it increasingly difficult to get there. This is largely due to a shortage of breath but also to the cramp-like pain in his legs which increases the further he walks.

The district nurse has been treating an ulcer on the top of his right foot, where his shoe had rubbed him, for the past 18 months without any success. He now seems to have pain in his legs most of the time, even at night when the only way of relieving it is by holding his legs over the end of the bed. During the week-end Jack was only able to walk downstairs and sit in the armchair as his foot was too painful to put on the ground. On Monday morning when the nurse visited, she realized the severity of his condition and called the general practitioner, who admitted him to hospital straight away.

On admission to hospital, Jack was found to have a haemoglobin concentration of 9.6 g/dl and a temperature of 38.4°C. His foot around the ulcer was red and shiny, his toes were cold to the touch. He complained of pain in the ulcer bed on touch, became very agitated when the nurse tried to dress it and demanded a cigarette. The nurse, who was very busy and had several new admissions to the ward, replied that if he didn't stop smoking he would have to have his leg off.

Aetiology

An arterial ulcer is the result of atherosclerosis of the lower arterial system and is often a progressive disease that can go unchecked for many years. Patients may complain of intermittent claudication, (pain on walking), ischaemic rest pain (pain often coming on at night when in bed) or episodes of critical limb ischaemia (requires prompt vascular attention). The condition will usually be accompanied by other circulatory disorders such as hypertension, cerebral vascular accidents and myocardial infarctions. One third of patients who present with ulceration will have critical limb ischaemia (Fox et al 1996).

Arterial ulcers are usually found on the distal parts of the digits, over bony prominences and the dorsum of the foot. They are often caused by friction from shoes or infection from bunions and corns.

Prognosis

The prognosis and outlook are often bleak if surgical intervention is not indicated. Claudication generally is treated conservatively with medication, advice on smoking cessation, diet and exercise. Surgical intervention is offered when the patient cannot live with the condition due to the advancing severity (Fox et al 1996). Surgery can reconstruct the arteries of the lower limb, so restoring or improving the blood supply (Figure 9.15).

Vascular surgery

The restoration of blood supply to the lower limb can involve a wide range of surgical procedures. For patients with isolated proximal stenotic or occlusive arterial lesions (often diabetic patients), percutaneous transluminal angioplasty (PTA) is a useful, minimally invasive procedure which entails the insertion of a balloon catheter into the vascular lumen of a major artery (the iliac or femoral artery). The deflated end of the catheter is placed at the site where the stenosis occurs. When in position, the balloon is inflated and stretches the vessel to enlarge the vascular lumen, so increasing blood flow distally.

Revascularization is achieved in 70% of patients with bypass surgery using synthetic or autogenous vein grafts to replace the conduit between proximal and distal arteries, so bypassing the diseased part of the artery (Fox et al 1996).

For the reconstruction of larger arteries, synthetic graft material can be used as the blood flow is rapid. However, the further distally the damage, the smaller the artery involved and microsurgical techniques using an autogenous graft are preferred. Figure 9.15b shows the various options for revascularizing the lower limb.

Assessment

Assessment of the affected limb includes (Clarke Maloney & Grace 2004):

- history (typically includes leg pain brought on by exercise and night pain, relieved by holding the limb in a dependent position)
- performing a physical examination to identify perfusion and reduced body heat
- Doppler assessment to determine ABPI
- examining the wound bed (ulcer has a punched-out appearance), particularly for the presence of devitalized tissue and infection
- identifying the presence of cellulitis related to severe infection.

Patients with vascular disease require urgent referral to a vascular surgeon for a full assessment of the extent of the disease. Treatment may include

Figure 9.15
(a) Arterial anatomy of a normal limb. (b) Surgical options for revascularizing the lower limb.

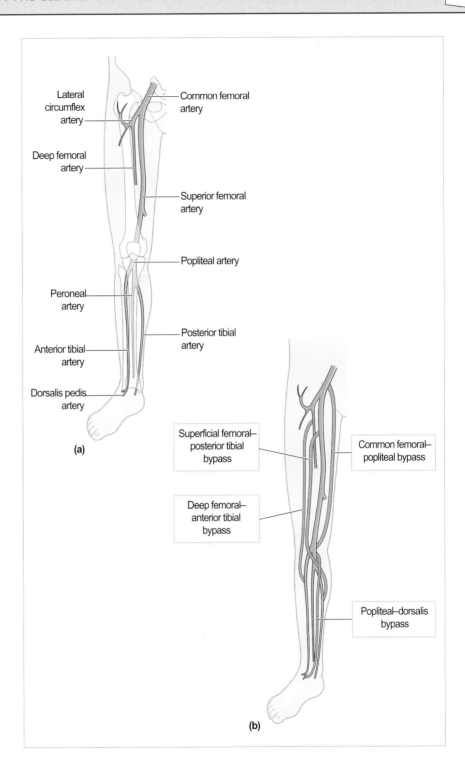

Lateral circumflex artery

Common femoral artery

Deep femoral artery

Superior femoral artery

Popliteal artery

Peroneal artery

Posterior tibial artery

Anterior tibial artery

Dorsalis pedis artery

(a)

Superficial femoral–posterior tibial bypass

Common femoral–popliteal bypass

Deep femoral–anterior tibial bypass

Popliteal–dorsalis bypass

(b)

angioplasty or reconstructive surgery. Revascularization has been achieved in some limbs with the use of thrombolytic therapy (agents such as urokinase, streptokinase and Cilostazol®) which has consequently led to healing of the arterial ulcer (Hickey 1994, Zolli 2004).

Management

The principles of managing patients with arterial ulceration are control of the symptoms and observation for deterioration of either the ulcer or the limb. The prognosis for healing can be poor which is demoralizing for both patient and nurse.

Local wound management

The nurse should be alert for deterioration in the wound bed involving tissue necrosis and the presence of wound infection. Retention bandages are used merely to keep the dressing in place and not to provide compression. Ensuring that the wound bed is given the best possible chance to heal is achieved by removal of necrotic and sloughy tissue and minimizing the numbers of organisms that will cause infection. This has been referred to as 'wound bed preparation' and has in some areas of specialist practice become a framework for the management of chronic wounds (Falanga 2000). Within this framework, wound debridement plays a fundamental role but also the use of dressings impregnated with iodine or silver will reduce the bacterial burden on the ulcer bed.

Pain control

Pain will be a major problem for these patients, often causing sleep disorders and inability to comply with treatment plans as advice given by the nurse, e.g. such as taking exercise, will worsen pain (Hofman 1997). Pain should be assessed using a validated pain scale (European Wound Management Association 2002), which ensures that the patient's experience of their pain is taken into account. The patient should be monitored closely and in most cases referral to a specialist may be warranted to ensure adequate pain control is achieved.

Psychological support

These patients may need a great deal of psychological support as the effect chronic ulceration has on an individual's quality of life is enormous. Awareness of the problems associated with vascular disease and the possibility of losing part or all of a limb requires a sensitive approach. Fortunately nurses and other health professionals now take into account the patient's perspective in order to gain an understanding of outcomes that are important to that individual (Roe et al 1995). Previously any type of leg ulceration was viewed as an inevitable part of growing old and problems such as odour and ulcer pain were considered to be something old people had to endure. Although healing would presumably be the preferred outcome, in the absence of any real potential to heal, relief of pain and the ability to have a good night's sleep are much more important. Measurement of the patient's quality of life has been the subject of much research in recent years and is now considered to be an essential element of ongoing assessment (Barrett & Teare 2000, Price and Harding 2000).

Nursing model for Jack

Besides the arterial problem that makes wound healing difficult in this patient's case, the nurse has to consider a model that will enlist the patient's cooperation otherwise he will not comply with any of the suggested treatments. Unfortunately his hospital admission did not set off on the right footing and much skill will be required to enlist the patient's trust in the staff and the system. Peplau's model emphasizes the interpersonal relationship between the nurse and patient and how it must develop in order for the patient's condition to improve.

The developmental models emphasize re-establishment of a developmental stage from which the individual has regressed. Intervention in these models often focuses on the educative-counselling role of the nurse which is likely to be of more importance in this case than actual treatment of the ulcer. Using Peplau's SOAP structure, try to identify a plan of care. For example:

S – complains of pain in his calf and foot, has no appetite for food, desperate for cigarettes

O – ulcer bed red and bleeding to touch, area around ulcer erythematous, patient looks pale and thin, troublesome cough

A – ulcer showing clinical signs of infection, temperature 38.4°C, haemoglobin level 9.6 g/dl, pneumoconiosis exacerbated by smoking 20–25 cigarettes a day

P – goal is eradication of infection, take swab to identify infecting organism, prescribe appropriate systemic antibiotics, use of impregnated low-adherent dressings.

PRACTICE POINTS

■ As Jack has an infection that needs to be treated, the problems initially identified are those of a physical nature. This is in line with Peplau's philosophy that the first purpose of the nurse is to help the patient to survive. The nurse can also make a significant difference to the amount of pain Jack is experiencing if the infection is treated correctly. This can form a basis on which a trusting relationship can develop. However, to build upon the nurse–patient relationship, it is essential to identify the psychosocial problems that are affecting his quality of life.

■ Maybe the nurse voiced Jack's underlying fear, i.e. that of losing his leg.

■ Continue working on this care plan, identifying problems and goals and planning the appropriate care.

FUNGATING MALIGNANT WOUNDS

The psychological problems of fungating malignant lesions, as described in Case study 9.3, can be as great as the physical problems.

Case study 9.3

Fungating malignant wounds

Mrs Dorothy Phillips is a 73-year-old retired nurse who was admitted to a hospice for management of a fungating carcinoma of her left breast. Although aware of changes in the shape of her breast some four years ago, Dorothy chose to ignore it until finally, prompted by her husband, she went to her general practitioner a year ago. By this time she was having discharge from the nipple and the surrounding skin had the characteristic *peau d'orange* (orange peel) appearance. As Dorothy and her worried husband had feared, she had a large tumour underneath her nipple which had progressed so extensively that surgery was not recommended. Following a short course of chemotherapy and radiotherapy, both Mr and Mrs Phillips and her oncologist decided that aggressive treatment was too physically and mentally distressing and that she would prefer palliative treatment only.

On admission to the hospice, it was found that the whole area of Dorothy's left breast was covered with fungating, malodorous, sloughy tissue. The malignancy had extended throughout the breast and into the lymphatic system, causing extensive lymphoedema of her left arm and leaving it immobilized.

Dorothy was fairly cheerful, although tired and anxious to return home as soon as possible. She was aware of her prognosis but was reluctant to discuss it openly. She was very distressed by advancing disease so evident in the wound. The odour was upsetting her and she was anxious that something should be done to keep the smell at bay, as she was embarrassed when visitors came to call. While she was at home her husband had, with the district nurse's assistance, been dressing the wound but it now required changing three or four times a day due to the constant leakage of exudate. She was not in any undue pain from the tumour but was becoming increasingly short of breath due to secondary deposits in her lung.

Aetiology

The incidence of fungating and ulcerating lesions is most commonly associated with breast cancer in women (Figure 9.16) although the true incidence of fungating malignant wounds is unknown (Grocott 1995a). Figures are based on estimations and are largely confined to the incidence of breast lesions (Ivetic & Lyne 1990, Thomas 1992).

Thomas (1992) identified the percentage and location of fungating wounds that were treated by specialist centres, as shown in Table 9.5.

The term 'fungating' is used to describe a malignancy which has ulcerated and infiltrated through the epithelium (Mortimer 1998). Carville (1995) describes a fungating lesion as one that results in a 'protruding growth' and ulceration as a cancerous growth that results in crater or cavity formation. Lesions infiltrate the epithelium and supporting lymph and blood vessels and, as the tumour extends, capillaries rupture, leading to tissue hypoxia, breakdown and necrosis. The accumulation of aerobic and anaerobic bacteria at the

Figure 9.16
A fungating malignant tumour of the left breast.

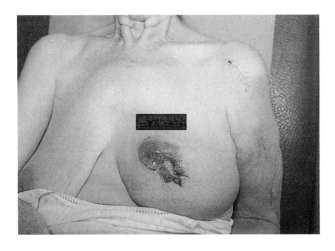

Table 9.5
Wound location in patients with fungating tumours undergoing treatment in specialist centres (reproduced with kind permission from Thomas 1992).

Location of wound	Percentage of total
Breast	62
Head/face	24
Groin/genitals	3
Back	3
Others	8

wound site causes the characteristic odour and exudate that make management of these wounds a challenge (Grocott 1995a). Bleeding may also be ever present due to either fragile capillary walls or infiltration of the tumour mass into surrounding blood vessels (Regnard & Tempest 1998).

Management

Improvement in the quality of life of patient and family can be achieved by alleviating the distressing symptoms of pain, infection, bleeding, malodour and discharge (Dunlop 1998). This was an area that had not been extensively explored until Grocott's work investigated ways of using the principles of modern wound management to create a conceptual framework for care (Grocott 2000).

It is essential to maintain the patient's dignity and self-esteem by supporting both carers and patient in care of the lesion by adopting a positive outlook to management. Patients may be considered incurable once skin ulceration is present, even without metastases. When treatment with curative intent is no longer appropriate or effective, carers must attempt to improve the quality of life and adopt a positive approach to topical management of the lesion.

Radiotherapy

Radiotherapy is usually well tolerated, even by the elderly, and can be given with or without hormonal treatment when surgery is not an option. Radiotherapy can halt the spread of disease, allowing some healing at the margins when the tumour bulk has decreased. It will also produce amelioration of symptoms such as pain and excess exudate, thereby increasing the patient's quality of life (Dixon 2002). Erythema may result but this is usually temporary. Due to advanced techniques in the control and direction of radiation, cutaneous radionecrosis (radiation burns to the skin) are now rarely seen (Salisbury et al 2000).

Wound management

The practitioner's attitude, especially during dressing procedures, can greatly influence the patient's own attitude and acceptance of the disease (Grocott 2000).

Whereas physical symptoms can be controlled, the psychological effects of the pressure of advancing disease can be intensely distressing to patients, carers and relatives (Fairbairn 1993). Feelings may range from depression, shame and embarrassment, to rejection and revulsion (Van-Toller 1994).

Cleansing fungating and ulcerating wounds with antiseptics was orginally thought to inhibit bacterial proliferation and diminish the offensive smell of anaerobic infection. Generally this has been found to be ineffective, as most cleansing agents are inactivated by body fluids (Leaper et al 1987). As bleeding points can be easily disturbed, only gentle irrigation with warm water or saline should be undertaken to remove debris and old dressings.

Topical metronidazole is effective in reducing odour (Hampson 1996) and can be applied directly onto the fungating mass and covered. Other means of odour control have been achieved with the use of charcoal-impregnated dressings although the absorbency of such may not always be adequate. Topical metronidazole is particularly useful for controlling malodour in malignant fungating lesions as anaerobic organisms, usually *Bacteroides*, colonize these lesions. However, the smell of these tumours is likely to be due to a complex interaction between anaerobes and aerobic organisms (Bowler 1998).

Dressings

Dressings should fit the margins of the wound precisely to avoid leakage onto clothing and excoriation to the periwound area and the nurse should find effective methods of fixing the dressing in place. Patients get very distressed when extra padding has to be applied between scheduled dressing changes and when clothes become soiled (Grocott 2000). Periwound skin should be treated with extreme caution and the use of skin preparation should be considered.

Grocott (1995b) identified the following principles that can be applied to the management of any fungating wound and has since built upon this framework in more depth (Grocott 2000).

- The control of pain through maintenance of optimum humidity at the wound site by using dressings that do not adhere to the tumour.
- Facilitation of wound debridement with removal of excess exudate and toxic materials to prevent deterioration and control smell.
- Topical antibiotics to control odour when appropriate.
- Removal of dressings without trauma.
- Restoration of body symmetry through use of cavity dressings.
- Achievement of cosmetic acceptability, without the need for bulky secondary dressings.
- Control bleeding when it occurs by using haemostatic dressings.

Nursing model for Dorothy

Roy's adaptation model (Roy & Andrews 1999) has been described in other works (Chadderton 1986) and is a useful framework when nursing the terminally ill. As outlined in Chapter 6, Roy's model is consistent with the hospice philosophy, in that when active treatment is not possible, symptomatic relief will help patients adapt to their particular situations and allow them to come to terms with their illness. Try using this model to plan the care for Dorothy.

PRACTICE POINTS

Unlike Fiona Starr in Chapter 6, Dorothy Phillips may have adapted to her situation, although denial has been a major part of her response to her illness. With the visible advancement of her disease both she and her husband may need to adapt to this stimulus in a way that will give them an improved quality of life in the terminal stages.

SUMMARY

This chapter illustrates the importance of the nurse–patient relationship whether it concerns helping a patient to understand the nature of their wound or coming to terms with disfigurement. What important features do these clinical case studies highlight for the nurse to consider?

- Educator: helping the patient with venous disease understand the importance of compression therapy in the healing process.
- Counsellor: giving the patient with arterial disease the opportunity to express their fears regarding their disease process.
- Advocate: maintaining the dignity and self-esteem of the patient with fungating wounds.

Once you are familiar with these basic principles of wound management, the above roles will enable you to enhance your care to a higher level of specialism.

FURTHER READING

Bale S, Harding K, Leaper D 2000 An introduction to wounds. Emap Healthcare Ltd, London.

Beard J D 2000 Chronic lower limb ischaemia. In: Donnelly R, London N J M (eds) ABC of arterial and venous disease. BMJ Books, London.

Callam M J, Harper D R, Dale J J, Ruckley C V 1987 Arterial disease in chronic leg ulceration: an underestimated hazard? Lothian and Forth Valley Leg Ulcer Study. British Medical Journal 294: 929–931.

Dunlop R 1998 Cancer: palliative care. Springer, London.

Jeffcoate W, Macfarlane R 1996 The diabetic foot: an illustrated guide to management. Chapman and Hall Medical, London.

Ruckley C V, Fowkes F G R, Bradbury A W (eds) 1998 Venous disease: epidemiology, management and delivery of care. Springer-Verlag, New York.

Stami S K, Shields J H, Sairr J H, Coleridge Smith P D 1992 Leg ulceration in venous disease. Postgraduate Medical Journal 68: 779–785.

REFERENCES

Barrett C, Teare J A 2000 Quality of life in leg ulcer assessment: patient's coping mechanisms. British Journal of Community Nursing 5(11): 530–540.

Bosanquet N 1992 Cost of venous ulcers: from maintanence therapy to investment programmes. Phlebology 1 (suppl): 44–46.

Bowler P 1998 The anaerobic and aerobic microbiology of wounds: a review. Wounds 10(6): 170–178.

Browse N L 1983 Venous ulceration. British Medical Journal 286: 1920–1922.

Burnand K G, Clemenson G, Whimster I, Browse N L 1976 Proceedings: extravascular fibrin deposition in response to venous hypertension – the cause of venous ulcers. British Journal of Surgery 63 8: 660–661.

Callam M J 1999 Leg ulcers and chronic venous insufficiency in the community. In: Ruckley C V, Fowkes F G R, Bradbury A W (eds) Venous disease: epidemiology, management and delivery of care. Springer-Verlag, New York.

Callam M J, Ruckley C V, Harper D R, Dale J J 1985 Chronic ulceration of the leg: extent of the problem and provision of care. British Medical Journal 290: 1855–1856.

Carville K 1995 Caring for cancerous wounds in the community. Journal of Wound Care 4(2): 46–48.

Chadderton H 1986 A stress adaptation model in terminal care. In: Kershaw B, Salvage J (eds) Models for nursing. John Wiley, Chichester.

Clarke Maloney M, Grace P 2004 Understanding the underlying causes for leg ulceration. Journal of Wound Care 13 (6): 215–218.

Coleridge-Smith P D, Thomas P, Scurr J H, Dormandy J A 1988 Causes of venous ulceration: a new hypothesis. British Medical Journal (Clinical Research) 296(6638): 1726–1727.

Cullum N 1994 The nursing management of leg ulcers in the community: a critical review of research. University of Liverpool, Department of Nursing, Liverpool.

Dixon J M 2002 ABC of breast diseases, 2nd edn. BMJ Books, London.

Dunlop R 1998 Cancer: palliative care. Springer, London.

European Wound Management Association 2002 Position document: pain at wound dressing changes. Medical Education Partnerships, London.

Fairbairn K 1993 Towards better care for women: understanding fungating breast lesions. Professional Nurse 9(3): 204–212.

Falanga V 2000 Classifications for wound bed preparation and stimulation of chronic wounds. Wound Repair and Regeneration 8(5): 347–352.

Finnie A 2002 Bandages and bandaging techniques for compression therapy. British Journal of Community Nursing 7 (3): 134–142.

Fletcher A 1992 The epidemiology of two common age-related wounds. Journal of Wound Care 1(4): 39–43.

Fox A D, Budd J S, Horrocks M 1996 Chronic lower limb arterial disease. Surgery 14(4): 82–88.

Grocott P 1995a The palliative management of fungating malignant wounds. Journal of Wound Care 4(5): 240–242.

Grocott P 1995b Assessment of fungating malignant wounds. Journal of Wound Care 4(7): 333–335.

Grocott P 2000 The palliative management of fungating malignant wounds. Journal of Wound Care 9(1): 4–16.

Hampson J P 1996 The use of metronidazole in the treatment of malodorous wounds. Journal of Wound Care 5(9): 421–425.

Hickey N C 1994 Drugs and peripheral vascular disease. Surgery 12(12): 271–274.

Hofman D 1997 Assessing and managing pain in leg ulcers. Community Nurse 3(6): 40–43.

Ivetic O, Lyne P A 1990 Fungating and ulcerationg malignant lesions: a review of the literature. Journal of Advanced Nursing 15(1): 83–88.

Leaper D, Cameron S, Lancaster J 1987 Antiseptic solutions. Community Outlook 83(14): 30–34.

Lindsay E 2001 Compliance with science: benefits of developing community Leg Clubs. British Journal of Nursing 10(22): S66–S74.

Mayberry J C, Mopneta G L, Taylor L M et al 1991 Fifteen year results of ambulatory compression therapy for chronic venous ulcers. Surgery 109: 575–581.

Moffatt C 2004 Factors that affect concordance with compression therapy. Journal of Wound Care 13(7): 291–294.

Morison M, Moffatt C 1994 A colour guide to the assessment and management of leg ulcers, 2nd edn. Mosby, London.

Mortimer P S 1998 Management of skin problems: medical aspects. In: Doyle D, Hanks G W C, MacDonald N (eds) Oxford textbook of palliative medicine, 2nd edn. Oxford University Press, Oxford.

NHS Centre for Reviews and Dissemination 1997 Compression therapy for venous leg ulcers. Effective Health Care Bulletin 3 (4): 1–12.

Price P, Harding K G 2000 Acute and chronic wounds: differences in self-reported health related quality of life. Journal of Wound Care 9(2): 93–95.

Regnard C F, Tempest S 1998 A guide to symptom relief in advanced cancer, 4th edn. Hochland and Hochland, Cheshire.

Riehl J P 1980 The Riehl interaction model. In: Riehl J P, Roy C (eds) Conceptual models for nursing practice. Appleton-Century-Crofts, New York.

Roe B, Cullum N, Hamer C 1995 Patients perspectives on chronic leg ulceration. In: Cullum N, Roe B (eds) Leg ulcers: nursing management. Scutari Press, London.

Roy C, Andrews H 1999 The Roy adaptation model, 2nd edn. Appleton and Lange, Stamford, Connecticut.

Royal College of Nursing (RCN) 1998 Clinical practice guidelines: the management of patients with venous leg ulcers. RCN, London.

Salisbury J R C, Anderson T J, Morgan D A 2000 ABC of breast diseases: breast cancer. British Medical Journal 321: 745–750.

Thomas S 1992 Current practices in the management of fungating lesions and radiation damaged skin. Surgical Materials Testing Laboratory, Bridgend General Hospital, Mid-Glamorgan.

Van-Toller S 1994 Invisible wounds: the effects of skin ulcer malodours. Journal of Wound Care 3 (2): 103–105.

Zolli A 2004 Foot ulceration due to arterial ulceration: role of cilostazol. Journal of Wound Care 13 (2): 45–47.

Evaluation

CHAPTER

10

Ways of evaluating care

KEY ISSUES   This chapter outlines different ways in which patient care can be measured and evaluated. Four main areas are considered.

■ Evaluation of the wound:
  wound measurement techniques
  prediction of healing
■ Evaluation of the delivery of care:
  clinical governance and audit
  guidelines
  standard setting
■ Evaluation of the patient:
  quality of life research
■ Evaluation of the nurse:
  role of the nurse specialist

INTRODUCTION   With increasing demands from the government and the general public for successful and measurable outcomes, methods of evaluating care are now a central focus of modern wound management. Clinical audit is an integral part of clinical governance that provides practitioners with the means to monitor and evaluate the quality of wound care a patient receives.

Of course, the method of evaluation will depend on what is being evaluated. Some outcomes will be easier to measure than others; for example, it is straightfoward to evaluate if a wound has healed when skin integrity is achieved but emotional healing of a wound caused by a burn or similar traumatic injury will be difficult to quantify. There is more interest now in subjective outcomes such as the patient's quality of life, especially for patients living with chronic wounds such as leg ulcers. Wound measurement on a regular basis can determine the rate of healing and can be used to evaluate if progress is being achieved according to the plan of management.

As outlined earlier, goals and outcomes should be set with evaluation in mind; use of subjective terminology will be difficult to evaluate and tells us nothing about the patient's care.

Figure 10.1
Determination of wound surface area (reproduced with kind permission from Flanagan 2003).

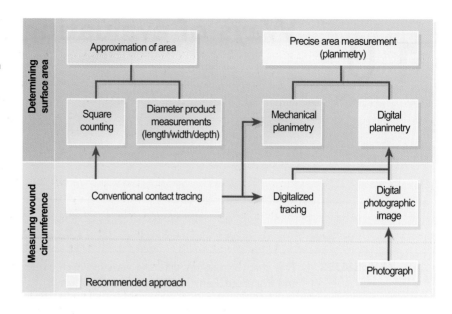

Table 10.1
Wound measurement techniques

Contact	Non-contact
Tracing overlays	Structured light
Depth gauges	Laser triangulation
Moulding material	Photogrammetry
Liquids	Stereophotogrammetry
Surface contour tracings	Monte Carlo technique
Ultrasound	Magnetic resonance imaging

EVALUATION OF THE WOUND

A number of methods have been described to assess wound size ranging from the very simple to very sophisticated and expensive systems (Figure 10.1). The purpose of these methods is to monitor the progress of healing from area or volume measurements. The different methods are usually described as contact or non-contact (Table 10.1), referring to whether there is physical contact with the wound (Plassmann 1995, Plassmann & Peters 2001).

In order to be used in everyday routine, methods need to be simple, quick and accurate otherwise they will not get integrated into practice. Most nurses tend to use contact measurements, such as tracing overlays, in one form or another. These tend to be unreliable as they give only a two-dimensional reading and often discrepancies between measurement of the same wound have been observed when different nurses are taking readings (Anthony 1993, Plassman et al 1994). They also have the disadvantages of the risk of wound contamination and discomfort for the patient on painful wounds (Plassman & Peters 2001). A simple and quick system of contact tracing (Visitrak®) has recently become available which on initial studies appears to give accurate measurement of wound area and circumference without such problems (Keast et al 2004).

Other methods such as filling the wound with saline to compare the amount of liquid the wound holds on each occasion (Berg et al 1990) or using dental moulding material (Resch et al 1988) are time-consuming and generally not suited to everyday practice.

Non-contact methods that give three-dimensional readings are proving to be a more sensitive measure of both area and volume. Techniques, such as structured light measurement called MAVIS (Plassman & Jones 1998), which gives an accurate picture of wound depth, have been experimentally developed but tend to be restricted to research settings. Digital cameras are now used more and more in routine practice and have been shown to be as accurate as contact tracing (Samad et al 2002). These can be used alongside computer programs which will analyse scanned transparency tracings or images taken by digital cameras with great accuracy (Flanagan 2003, Plassman & Peters 2001). As it requires the use of a computer loaded with specialized software this can present limitations in terms of both cost and space for many areas of clinical practice. Other sophisticated systems for wound volume measurement include stereophotogrammetry and scanning laser systems (Langemo et al 1998).

An important limitation that is common to all methods is deciding where the edge of the wound lies. This affects the accuracy of the techniques and in particular interobserver accuracy (Langemo et al 1998, Plassman and Peters 2001).

Complex measures are not available to all practitioners and the simpler contact measurements, although less reliable, may be the best choice available at the present time to the vast majority dealing with wounds.

Prediction of healing

Although it is known that complete healing involves all underlying structures and tissue, for most practitioners healing is said to be achieved when the wound has epithelialized. Different wound types have varying times to healing but the factors that influence this rate of healing, particularly in chronic wounds, are still not entirely clear. Researchers are now attempting to investigate and identify the key factors that will enable practitioners to predict in advance the likely outcome and therefore the most appropriate treatment for the wound.

From work done to date on patients with venous leg ulcers, it would appear that the initial size of the ulcer and the length of time the ulcer has been present are two key predictors of the probability of healing within a certain time frame (Kantor & Margolis 1998, Margolis et al 2004).

The methods used to produce this information are related to complex statistical analysis on large groups of patients. Although confined at present to work carried out in specialist research centres, this will undoubtedly become a valuable basis for routine assessment of the patient's wound-healing potential for all practitioners in the future.

EVALUATING DELIVERY OF CARE

The demand for evidence-based practice and a greater public expectation for quality health service have required practitioners to become focused on providing clinically effective care. Since 1997 the government has produced a set of policies, programmes and structures to put the patient at the centre of service planning and delivery. In 1999 the NHS Plan introduced a range of measures to raise quality and address unacceptable variations in service delivery. Clinical governance became the heart of the provision of quality care and the development of the Commission for Health Improvement (CHI), charged with reviewing the measures taken by trusts to introduce clinical governance processes, was seen as a major step foward.

> Clinical effectiveness is about doing the right thing in the right way for the right patient at the right time. (RCN 1996).

Clinical audit

When changes are made in practice to improve clinical effectiveness, it is essential that a mechanism is in place to check that the changes are being implemented and confirm if the change is beneficial or requires still further improvement to enhance the quality of care. This mechanism is referred to as clinical audit and lies at the heart of the clinical governance process. It is defined as: '. . . a quality improvement process that seeks to improve patient care and outcomes through systematic review of care against explicit criteria and the implementation of change' (NICE 2002).

Ideally audit should be multidisciplinary but in general it is carried out by doctors and nurses. It should focus on the patient, aiming to improve clinical effectiveness and therefore the quality of care the patient receives. Audits can be carried out retrospectively after care has been given or prospectively while the patient is being cared for.

Audit may be done at random, without any change in practice being made, or linked to standard setting where criteria relating to the standard can be measured in the audit.

Thankfully, with the introduction of NICE guidelines, standards and criteria by which care can be measured are now available in some aspects of wound care. These are based on a review of the literature and graded according to strength of evidence (see Appendix). However, there is a problem in the implementation of audit practices in wound care in that there is still a scarcity of sound evidence to support a large amount of wound care.

Various methods of data collection can be used such as interviews of patients and examination of case notes. However, as with any form of data collection, principles of ethics and confidentiality need to be maintained.

Following completion of audit, where findings show good practice this should be fed back to those concerned. If there are problems in practice, a thorough investigation should be carried out and a detailed plan of action implemented in order to bring about improvements in care (see Figure 10.2).

Guidelines

One way of ensuring clinical effectiveness and the implementations of evidence-based practice has been via the production of clinical guidelines. Their usage in the UK began with the establishment of clinical audit, as guidelines were able to define standards by which care could be measured (Andrews & Redmond 2004). With the increasing demand for evidence-based medicine and the setting up of institutions such as NICE who were charged with the responsibility for guidelines, clinical guidelines have become a familiar part of clinical practice both in the UK and beyond (Woolf et al 1999).

Guidelines for the management of patients with wounds may be considered to be useful in an area where, formulated properly, they should eliminate inappropriate and costly treatments (McGuckin et al 1996).

Figure 10.2
The clinical audit process (reproduced with kind permission from *Nursing Times* 1998).

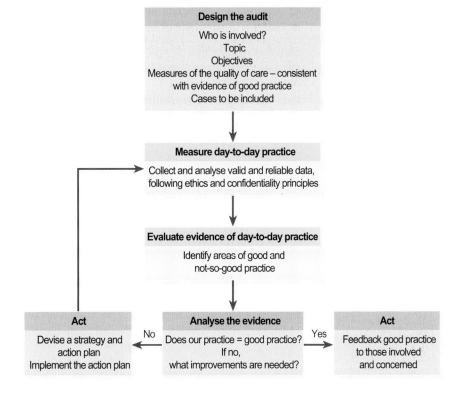

Rapid expansion of the development of sophisticated dressings means that unit costs of dressings also rise and decision making may be dictated by ritualistic practice rather than by appropriate research-based evidence. With the production of national guidelines, many trusts have realized the benefit of using them as a basis for cost-effective wound care protocols which are linked to hospital formularies.

Advantages of guidelines (RCN 1997)
- Reduce unacceptable or undesirable variations in clinical practice.
- Offer a way of implementing research findings.
- Provide a focus for discussion among both health professionals and patients/clients.
- Help professionals from different disciplines come to an agreement about treatment.
- Provide a quality framework against which to measure practice.
- Offer valuable information for use by those bidding for resources.
- Help those who commission and purchase care to make informed decisions.
- Give managers useful data for assessing treatment costs.

Disadvantages of guidelines
- They can be wrong, based on anecdotal evidence rather than scientific fact.
- Only a small amount of wound care has been tested in well-designed studies and it can be difficult to formulate evidence-based guidelines (Woolf et al 1999).

- Difficult to disseminate, especially at a local level (Russell & Grimshaw 1992).
- Difficult to persuade experienced practitioners that they need them.

However, guidelines should not be used to replace individual accountability. Clinical guidelines cannot be used to mandate, authorize or outlaw treatment options (Hurwitz 1999).

However robust, guidelines need to be interpreted sensibly and applied with discretion. Practitioners should interpret their application by taking into account local circumstances and the needs and wishes of individual patients.

Standards in wound care

Whereas there were few standards in wound care in the 1990s, this problem has largely disappeared due to the introduction of NHS national standards which have been produced by the Department of Health, National Service Frameworks (NSFs), NICE Guidelines or NHS Essence of Care benchmark statements (see Appendix).

Why set standards?

Setting standards can help to provide an acceptable level of care to patients and carers. Considered to be part of a package that leads to quality, standards and associated criteria can specify what is to be measured and used as a means of evaluating the level of care given.

How do we know that the standards set are acceptable to our patients and to other colleagues? Everybody has individual standards. Standards that we set ourselves, and on which we base the way we live, will have been largely influenced by our cultural and environmental background.

Within a professional organization such as nursing, certain standards will have been set and nurses are expected to conform to them on becoming part of the profession, but even these standards change according to the social and cultural norms of the environment. For example, it was standard practice in nursing in the 1970s to address patients by their surname and title (Mrs, Mr, etc.) and to refer to colleagues as 'Sister', 'Staff Nurse' or 'Doctor'. This practice reflected aspects of life outside nursing. This standard has now changed to a less formal approach, with patients and staff often calling each other by their first names. This may be seen by some as a lowering of standards, especially for nurses who trained in the era when last names only were used. This is a subjective type of standard which refers to a person's attitude or belief and it is difficult to measure whether it affects the quality of care given.

Standards that directly affect the level of care given are concerned with knowledge (evidence) and skills (competency). For example, it is generally accepted that inadequate hand washing is a major source of cross infection and leads to a higher incidence of wound infection. A hospital may have set a standard such as 'postoperative wound infection will be no higher than 5%'. Nurses may accept this as a hospital standard but lack the knowledge of the mechanisms of cross infection or the skills of performing adequate hand washing. It is therefore of vital importance that these things are considered when standards are introduced into practice, otherwise they will not be achieved. The introduction of clinical audit has helped tremendously as it will identify the reasons why a standard such as this is not being met.

Advantages of setting standards

Written standards allow practice to be critically examined. It is a way of bringing theory and practice together and highlights where resources, knowledge and skills are lacking.

As in the example of cross contamination and wound infection given above, it could be assumed that all nurses know about correct hand-washing technique and its role in prevention of postoperative infection. However, it was only when this standard statement was formulated that these two key factors were addressed by the introduction of an educational programme on infection control.

Standard setting gives nurses and other professionals an opportunity to identify what they are trying to achieve and discover whether they achieve it.

Disadvantages of setting standards

Standards are often accused of being a statement of the obvious and are seen as a paper exercise. Many practitioners do not see the benefit of written standards as they are convinced that their personal standard of care is good enough and that they maintain a consistently high standard of care at all times. This may well be true of many individuals involved in providing care but there is no proof to support this belief and they may be totally ignorant of the potential harm this practice may cause. Again, clinical audit will identify discrepancies in practice and provide objective proof of the problems to those concerned.

In order to implement national standards, many trusts have developed local protocols or integrated care pathways. Where there are no national standards, the best available evidence will be used to formulate the standards.

All the above methods tell us about the care we give as nurses in terms of objective, measurable outcomes. The traditional evaluation of medical or nursing treatments has been through quantitative measurements of healing rates or reduction in morbidity. An area that has been ignored until recently is how the patient feels and what psychosocial problems affect the patient's day-to-day living. Quality of life research is now directed at trying to quantify the subjective experiences of these patients.

EVALUATING THE PATIENT'S QUALITY OF LIFE

The term 'quality of life' is often used freely among health professionals with the assumption that everybody has the same understanding of what it refers to.

Quality of life is such a broad concept and is so subjective that many clinicians still question its relevance or validity to a patient's outcome.

It is unlikely that all medical treatments would be able to improve the true quality of a person's life, including job prospects and living accommodation. However, most nurses would like to think that they are able to improve their patients' quality of life by maintaining a good standard of nursing care.

The definition of what constitutes a good quality of life will vary between individuals but in today's health care, it has become part of a holistic view of the individual within health-care systems. Definitions now centre around 'health-related quality of life' (HRQoL) outcomes, which refer to not only the impact of health and illness on physical and social functioning but also psychological well-being. This ensures that data are collected on both objective functioning and subjective well-being.

Fallowfield (1990), a psychologist, defined four areas or core domains, of which psychological factors were placed first.

- Psychological
  depression
  anxiety
  adjustment or illness
- Social
  personal and sexual relationships
  engagement in social and leisure activities
- Occupational
  ability and desire to carry out paid employment
  ability to cope with household duties
- Physical
  pain
  mobility
  sleep
  appetite and nausea
  sexual functioning

The order of these core domains may be rearranged according to the individual's professional background, e.g. a nurse may list the physical or social domain as being of greater importance, whereas a social worker would probably consider occupational needs.

It can be argued that nurses have already identified these as important aspects of a patient's overall quality of life, given that most nursing models address these core areas in their assessment framework. But one important question should also be addressed: 'Who will assess changes in life quality?'. Researchers agree that the patient is the best person to rate their own lives but if the patient is unable to complete such an assessment, the nurse will have to identify problems, which can prove difficult.

Also once identified, how can they be evaluated to demonstrate a significant improvement to the patient's quality of life? As it is such a difficult area to define and measure, researchers have attempted to create standardized tests using a psychometric approach (Price et al 1994).

Psychometric tests   Psychometry uses standardized tests to measure any given concept (Price & Harding 1993). These include generic health scales and disease-specific scales. Generic tests cover a wide range of domains and are very useful for making comparisons in terms of functional improvement across conditions and diseases, the most widely used being the Nottingham Health Profile (Hunt et al 1989) and the SF-36 Health Survey.

Disease-specific measures investigate the impact of a specific condition in terms of the symptoms related to that condition; such tools may be more sensitive to changes over time which are related to the condition. Disorders such as diabetes mellitus (Wallymahmed et al 1991) and chronic pain (Chibnall & Tait 1990) are earlier examples.

The decision as to which test will effectively evaluate the patient's quality of life will depend on the type of patient and wound under study and the particular research or clinical questions that needs to be answered. Previous authors have used a variety of established tests together to investigate quality of life in patients with leg ulcers (Franks et al 1994, Hamer et al 1994) as at that time there were no condition-specific measures for wounds. However, it is recognized that the use of general tools will not address specific problems and researchers have now developed condition-specific tools to assess the health-related quality of life in patients with leg ulcers and diabetic foot ulcers (Price & Harding 2004, Vileikyte et al 2003).

EVALUATING THE CONTRIBUTION OF THE SPECIALIST NURSE

So far we have looked at ways of evaluating the progress of the wound, the quality of care given and the patient's quality of life. Perhaps, finally, it is appropriate to look at the role of specialist nurses and evaluate their unique skills that can influence the overall care and management of the patient.

The clinical nurse specialist

The clinical nurse specialist is now a well-established part of the NHS whose contribution has clearly influenced the type of care patients with wounds can expect to receive (McGee & Castledine 2003). Although their role developed in North America in the 1960s (Storr 1988), it was not until the beginning of 1980 that posts were created in the UK.

Hamric and Spross (1989) previously defined the clinical nurse specialist as 'a registered nurse who, through study and supervised practice at a graduate level, has become an expert in a defined area of knowledge and practice in a selected clinical area of nursing'. Since this initial definition, many governmental and educational changes have occurred which have influenced the role, responsibilities and pay structures of specialist nurses. The introduction of the consultant nurse role (DoH 2000) and Agenda for Change (DoH 2003) and changes to the general practitioners' contract will during the next five years witness the strengthening or erosion of the nurse's role in the delivery of wound care.

Although all changes are concerted attempts to retain experienced nurses at the bedside, many nurses have struggled to be appointed as clinical nurse specialists or tissue viability nurses at appropriate grades and have had to make business cases to trusts to prove and demonstrate the benefit of the role (Coull 2004). This in part is due to the role of the clinical nurse specialist which can vary greatly, from that of tissue viability nurses, whose main area of specialism in some trusts is centred around pressure ulcer management and prevention, to leg ulcer specialists. Because of the disparity in roles and titles, often they can be working at almost any grade and it is often difficult to evaluate how effective such specialists are. This has become an area of concern for many nurses in such posts due to the evaluation of roles required for regrading under the Agenda for Change scheme (Maylor 2004).

The clinical nurse specialist has five commonly accepted major roles (Storr 1988), which still tend to be used as a basis for job descriptions as there is little standardization and regulation of clinical nurse specialists (McCreaddie 2001). However, under Agenda for Change (DoH 2003) these roles are clearly linked to education and clinical competences and should provide a framework to develop and enhance clinical nurse specialists and nurse consultant posts.

- Practitioner: carries out direct patient care.
- Teacher and educator: to patient, family, nursing staff, students.

- Consultant: plans and advises on total care with patient, family, nursing staff.
- Researcher: carries out research relevant to specialty.
- Change agent: acts as catalyst for change within the organization.

Consider these five roles in relation to a nurse specialist in wound care.

Practitioner

In carrying out direct patient care, the clinical nurse specialist can act as a role model for other practitioners with whom they are in contact.

Using their advanced knowledge of wound care, they are able to assess patients comprehensively using a nursing model where appropriate, while developing individual nursing care plans.

Their advanced nursing skills enable care to be delivered at a high level, setting the standard to be followed by those continuing the day-to-day nursing care of the patient.

Teacher and educator

Wound care specialists can disseminate knowledge among other practitioners, patients and carers in the clinical application of their work. Often they are responsible for setting up courses (Flanagan 1995, Jones et al 2004), clinics and link-nurse schemes. Professional groups such as the Tissue Viability Society, Wound Care Society and National Association of Tissue Viability Nurse Specialists (TVNA 2002), which are run and supported by specialist nurses, also contribute to the spread of knowledge as they provide peer support, organize study days and produce newsletters and journals.

Consultant

Psychological support of staff and patients is an essential aspect of the role of the clinical nurse specialist (Sparacino 2000). Often specialists will act as counsellors for staff and patients as they are seen as being approachable (McGee & Castledine 2003). It is vitally important, therefore, that individuals undertaking this role are easily accessible to both staff and patients.

Researcher

A major part of the specialist role is involvement in research. Conducting research trials or evaluating existing research constitutes a large part of the day-to-day work of the clinical nurse specialist. Nurses are often accused of not reading current research or transferring research findings into practice; the specialist can bridge this gap between theory and practice to the benefit of both nurse and patient .

Change agent

The specialist should act as a catalyst for change within the organization. However, change is often difficult to achieve but the specialist can overcome resistance by using communication skills and fostering relationships with medical and nursing staff. Seen to occupy a position of power and often viewed as having charismatic qualities (Storr 1988), the specialist can change ritualistic and outdated practices which are often detrimental to patient care (Sparacino 2000).

The benefits of specialist nursing

The above roles illustrate the qualities the wound care specialist is required to have and how they can be used in practice. Research has confirmed that expertise, further training and effective methods of organizing care are essential components of nursing that lead to improvement in the quality of patient care (Read 2003).

Where the clinical nurse specialist is perceived as a powerful clinical expert and is an accepted figure in the organization, then high-quality nursing practice is seen to be the result (Hamric et al 2000). The introduction of the nurse consultant post, that offers experienced clinical nurses a new career structure with better pay awards, seems the obvious step for existing the clinical nurse specialist or tissue viability nurse. However, there are clearly problems in differentiating between the two roles, particularly as these are linked to pay banding (Maylor 2004). Although at present there are very few nurse consultants in the UK, it is evident that there is a danger that this role may be further construed as medicalization of a fundamental aspect of nursing care.

Wound care specialists are increasing in number, as is the level of education available to them. To obtain a true evaluation of their effectiveness on the quality of care, further research and clinical audit must be continued.

PRACTICE POINT

If you work with wound care specialists, think of ways in which they improve the quality of care the patient receives.

SUMMARY

Evaluation of care can be achieved in many different ways. Each method concentrates on a particular aspect of wound care.

Evaluation should always be considered at the assessment and planning phase of management, not as an afterthought.

The main areas of evaluation can be summarized as follows.

- **Evaluation of the wound**
  Wound measurement techniques
  Prediction of healing
- **Evaluation of the delivery of care**
  Clinical audit
  Guidelines
  Standard setting
- **Evaluation of the patient**
  Quality of life
- **Evaluation of the nurse**
  Role of the specialist nurse in wound care

FURTHER READING

Bowling A 1997 Measuring health: a review of quality of life measurement scales, 2nd edn. Open University Press, Buckingham.

Bury T, Mead J 1998 Evidence-based healthcare: a practical guide for therapists. Heinemann, Oxford.

Hamric A B, Spross J A, Hanson C M (eds) 2000 Advanced nursing practice: an integrative approach. W B Saunders, Philadelphia.

Langemo D K, Melland H, Hanson D et al 1998 Two-dimensional wound measurement: comparison of four techniques. Advances in Wound Care 11: 337–343.

Luthert J M, Robinson L (eds) 1993 The Royal Marsden Hospital manual of standards of care. Blackwell Scientific, Oxford.

McGee P, Castledine G (eds) 2003 Advanced nursing practice, 2nd edn. Blackwell Scientific, Oxford.

REFERENCES

Andrews E J, Redmond H P 2004 A review of clinical guidelines. British Journal of Surgery 91: 956–964.

Anthony D 1993 Measuring pressure sores and venous leg ulcers. Community Outlook August: 35–36.

Berg W, Traneroth C, Gunnarsson A, Lossing C 1990 A method for measuring pressure sores. Lancet 335: 1445–1446.

Chibnall J T, Tait R C 1990 The quality of life scale: a preliminary study with chronic pain patients. Psychological Health 4: 283–292.

Coull A 2004 Editorial: how useful is the tissue viability nurse specialist? British Journal of Nursing 13(11): S3.

Department of Health 2000 The NHS Plan: a plan for improvement, a plan for reform. Stationery Office, London.

Department of Health 2003 Agenda for Change. Department of Health, London.

Fallowfield L 1990 The quality of life: the missing dimension in health care. Souvenir Press, London.

Flanagan M 1995 A contemporary approach to wound care education. Journal of Wound Care 4(9): 422–424.

Flanagan M 2003 Wound measurement: can it help monitor progression to healing? Journal of Wound Care 12 (5):189–194.

Franks P, Moffatt C, Connolly M et al 1994 Community leg ulcer clinics: effect on quality of life. Phlebology 9: 83–86.

Hamer C, Cullum N A, Rose B H 1994 Patients' perceptions of chronic leg ulceration. Journal of Wound Care 3(2): 99–101.

Hamric A B, Spross J A (eds) 1989 The clinical nurse specialist in theory and practice, 2nd edn. W B Saunders, Philadelphia.

Hamric A B, Spross J A, Hanson C M (eds) 2000 Advanced nursing practice: an intergrative approach. W B Saunders, Philadelphia.

Hunt S, McKenna S P, McEwan J 1989 The Nottingham Health Profile users' manual. Galen Research and Consultancy, Manchester.

Hurwitz B 1999 Legal and political considerations of clinical practice guidelines. British Medical Journal 318: 661–664.

Jones V J, Corbett J, Tarran N 2004 Postgraduate Diploma/Master of Science in Wound Healing and Tissue Repair. International Wound Journal 1(1): 38–41.

Kantor J, Margolis D 1998 Efficacy and prognostic value of simple wound measurements. Archives of Dermatology 134: 1571–1574.

Keast D, Bowering C K, Evans A W et al 2004 MEASURE: a proposed assessment framework for developing best practice recommendations for wound assessment. Wound Repair and Regeneration 12 (suppl): S1-S17.

Langemo D K, Melland H, Hanson D et al 1998 Two-dimensional wound measurement: comparison of four techniques. Advances in Wound Care 11: 337–343.

Margolis D, Allen-Taylor L, Hoffstad O et al 2004 The accuracy of venous leg ulcer prognostic models in a wound care system. Wound Repair and Regeneration 12: 163–168.

Maylor M 2004 Where will clinical nurse specialists be placed on Agenda for Change? British Journal of Nursing 13 (15): S26-S32.

McCreaddie M 2001 The role of the clinical nurse specialist. Nursing Standard 16: 33–38.

McGee P, Castledine G (eds) 2003 Advanced nursing practice, 2nd edn. Blackwell Publishing, Oxford.

McGuckin M, Stineman M, Goin J, Williams S 1996 The road to developing standards for the diagnosis and treatment of venous leg ulcers. Ostomy/Wound Management 42 (10A suppl): 62S-65S.

NICE 2002 Principles for best practice in clinical audit. Radcliffe Medical Press, Oxford.

Plassmann P 1995 Measuring wounds. Journal of Wound Care 4(6): 269–274.

Plassmann P, Jones T D 1998 MAVIS a non-invasive instrument to measuring area and volume of wounds. Medical Engineering and Physics 20 (5): 332–338.

Plassmann P, Peters M J 2001 Recording wound care effectiveness. Journal of Tissue Viability 12(1): 24–28.

Plassman P, Melhuish J, Harding K G 1994 Methods of measuring wound size: a comparative study. Wounds 6 (2): 54–61.

Price P E, Harding K G 1993 Defining quality of life. Journal of Wound Care 2(5): 304–306.

Price P E, Harding K G 2004 Cardiff Wound Impact Schedule: the development of a condition specific questionnaire to assess health related quality of life in patients with chronic wounds of the lower limb. International Wound Journal 1 (1): 10–17.

Price P E, Butterworth R J, Bale S, Harding K G 1994 Measuring quality of life in patients with granulating wounds. Journal of Wound Care 3(1): 49–50.

Read S 2003 Exploring role development and role expansion: is there a difference and does it matter? Proceedings of Consensus Conference, Royal College of Physicians, Edinburgh.

Resch C S, Kerner E, Robson M C et al 1988 Pressure sore volume measurement. Journal of the American Geriatric Society 36(5): 444–446.

Royal College of Nursing (RCN) 1996 Clinical effectiveness. A Royal College of Nursing guide. RCN, London.

Royal College of Nursing (RCN) 1997 Clinical guidelines: what you need to know. RCN, London.

Russell I T, Grimshaw J M 1992 The effectiveness of referral guidelines: a review of methods and findings of published evaluations. In: Roland M O, Coulter A (eds) Hospital referrals. Oxford University Press, Oxford.

Samad A, Hayes S, French L, Dodds S 2002 Digital imaging versus conventional contact tracing for the objective measurement of venous leg ulcers. Journal of Wound Care 11: 137–140.

Sparacino P 2000 The clinical nurse specialist. In: Hamric A B, Spross J A, Hanson C M (eds) Advanced nursing practice: an integrative approach. W B Saunders, Philadelphia.

Storr G 1988 The clinical nurse specialist: from the outside looking in. Journal of Advanced Nursing 13: 265–272.

Tissue Viability Nurses Association (TVNA) 2002 The Tissue Viability Nurses Association. Journal of Tissue Viability 12(1): 35.

Vileikyte L, Peyrot M, Bundy C et al 2003 The development and validation of a neuropathy and foot ulcer specific quality of life instrument. Diabetes Care 26 (9): 2549–2555.

Wallymahmed M E, Baker G A, Macfarlane I A 1991 Quality of life assessment in diabetes: a preliminary study of young adults in Liverpool. Practical Diabetes 9: 193–195.

Woolf S H, Grol R, Hutchinson A, Eccles M, Grimshaw J 1999 Potential benefits, limitations and harms of clinical guidelines. British Medical Journal 318: 527–530.

APPENDIX

Section of NICE (2003) Pressure Ulcer Prevention Cinical Guideline 7

The following guidance is evidence based. The recommendations in this document are derived from two clinical guidelines, *Pressure Ulcer Risk Assessment and Prevention and Clinical Practice Guideline for Pressure-relieving Devices: the Use of Pressure-relieving Devices (Beds, Mattresses and Overlays) for the Prevention of Pressure Ulcers in Primary and Secondary Care* (see Section 5), which use different grading schemes. In the guideline on pressure ulcer risk assessment and prevention, evidence grading was 1, 2 and 3; in the guideline on pressure-relieving devices, recommendations were graded A, B, C and D. The grading schemes arc described in Appendix A. Summaries of the evidence on which the guidance is based are provided in the full guidelines (see Section 5).

The guideline on pressure ulcer risk assessment and prevention was published in 2001*. Its recommendations have been incorporated into this document, but the evidence used to develop it was not reviewed or updated during the development of the guideline on pressure-relieving devices.

1 Guidance
The recommendations in this document are relevant to:

- those who are vulnerable to or at elevated risk of developing pressure ulcers
- families and carers
- healthcare professionals who share in caring for those who are vulnerable to or at elevated risk of developing pressure ulcers
- those with responsibility for purchasing pressure-relieving devices.

1.1   Risk assessment and prevention

1.1.1   Identifying individuals vulnerable to or at elevated risk of pressure ulcers

1.1.1.1   Assessing an individual's risk of developing pressure ulcers should involve both informal and formal assessment procedures.   **3**

1.1.1.2   Risk assessment should be carried out by personnel who have undergone appropriate training to recognise the risk factors that contribute to the development of pressure ulcers and know how to initiate and maintain correct and suitable preventative measures.   **3**

1.1.1.3   The timing of risk assessment should be based on each individual case. However, it should take place within 6 hours of the start of admission to the episode of care.   **3**

* The recommendations were published by NICE in April 2001: National Institute for Clinical Excellence (2001) Pressure ulcer risk management and prevention. *Inherited Clinical Guideline* B. London: National Institute for Clinical Excellence.

1.1.1.4 If an individual is considered not to be vulnerable to or at elevated risk of pressure ulcers on initial assessment, reassessment should occur if there is a change in an individual's condition that increases risk (see Section 1.1.3). **3**

1.1.1.5 All formal assessments of risk should be documented/recorded and made accessible to all members of the interdisciplinary team. **3**

1.1.2 Use of risk assessment tools

1.1.2.1 Risk assessment tools should only be used as an *aide memoire* and should not replace clinical judgment. **1**

1.1.3 Risk factors

1.1.3.1 An individual's potential to develop pressure ulcers may be influenced by the following intrinsic risk factors, which therefore should be considered when performing a risk assessment: **2**
- reduced mobility or immobility
- sensory impairment
- acute illness
- level of consciousness
- extremes of age **2**
- vascular disease
- severe chronic or terminal illness
- previous history of pressure damage
- malnutrition and dehydration.

1.1.3.2 The following extrinsic risk factors are involved in tissue damage and should be removed or diminished to prevent injury: pressure, shearing and friction. **2**

1.1.3.3 The potential of an individual to develop pressure ulcers may be exacerbated by the following factors, which therefore should be considered when performing a risk assessment: medication and moisture to the skin. **2**

1.1.4 Skin inspection

1.1.4.1 Skin inspection should occur regularly and the frequency determined in response to changes in the individual's condition in relation to either deterioration or recovery. **3**

1.1.4.2 Skin inspection should be based on an assessment of the most vulnerable areas of risk for each patient. These are typically: heels; sacrum; ischial tuberosities; parts of the body affected by anti-embolic stockings; femoral trochanters; parts of the body where pressure, friction or shear is exerted in the course of an individual's daily living activities; parts of the body where there are external forces exerted by equipment and/or clothing; elbows; temporal region of skull; shoulders; back of head and toes. **3**
Other areas should be inspected as necessitated by the patient's condition.

1.1.4.3   Individuals who are willing and able should be encouraged, following education, to inspect their own skin.   **3**

1.1.4.4   Individuals who are wheelchair users should use a mirror to inspect the areas that they cannot see easily or get others to inspect them.   **3**

1.1.4.5   Healthcare professionals should be aware of the following signs, which may indicate incipient pressure ulcer development: persistent erythema; non-blanching hyperaemia previously identified as non-blanching erythema; blisters; discolouration; localised heat; localised oedema and localised induration. In those with darkly pigmented skin: purplish/bluish localised areas of skin; localised heat that, if tissue becomes damaged, is replaced by coolness; localised oedema and localised induration.   **3**

1.1.4.6   Skin changes should be documented/recorded immediately.   **3**

1.2   Pressure ulcer prevention

1.2.1   Positioning

1.2.1.1   Individuals who are vulnerable to or at elevated risk of pressure ulcer development should be repositioned and the frequency of repositioning determined by the results of skin inspection and individual needs, not by a ritualistic schedule.   **3**

1.2.1.2   Repositioning should take into consideration other relevant matters, including the patient's medical condition, their comfort, the overall plan of care and the support surface.   **3**

1.2.1.3   Positioning of patients should ensure that: prolonged pressure on bony prominences is minimised, bony prominences are kept from direct contact with one another, and friction and shear damage is minimised.   **3**

1.2.1.4   A re-positioning schedule, agreed with the individual, should be recorded and established for each person vulnerable to pressure ulcers.   **3**

1.2.1.5   Individuals or carers, who are willing and able, should be taught how to redistribute weight.   **3**

1.2.1.6   Manual handling devices should be used correctly in order to minimise shear and friction damage. After manoeuvring, slings, sleeves or other parts of the handling equipment should not be left underneath individuals.   **3**

1.2.2   Seating

1.2.2.1   Seating assessments for aids and equipment (otherwise known as assistive technologies) should be carried out by trained assessors who have the acquired specific knowledge and expertise (for example, physiotherapists or occupational therapists).   **3**

1.2.2.2   Advice from trained assessors with acquired specific knowledge and expertise should be sought about correct seating positions.   **3**

1.2.2.3   Positioning of individuals who spend substantial periods of time in a chair or wheelchair should take into account distribution of weight, postural alignment and support of feet. **3**

1.2.2.4   The management of a patient in a sitting position is important. Even with appropriate pressure relief, it may be necessary to restrict sitting time to less than 2 hours until the condition of an individual with an elevated risk changes. **D**

1.2.2.5   No seat cushion has been shown to perform better than another, so this guideline makes no recommendation about which type to use for pressure redistribution purposes. **3**

1.2.3   Use of aids

1.2.3.1   The following should not be used as pressure-relieving aids: water-filled gloves; synthetic sheepskins*; doughnut-type devices. **3**

1.2.4   Pressure-relieving devices (beds, mattresses and overlays)

1.2.4.1   Decisions about which pressure-relieving device to use should be based on cost considerations and an overall assessment of the individual. Holistic assessment should include all of the following: **D**
   ■ identified levels of risk
   ■ skin assessment
   ■ comfort
   ■ general health state **D**
   ■ lifestyle and abilities
   ■ critical care needs
   ■ acceptability of the proposed pressure-relieving equipment to the patient and/or carer and should not be based solely on scores from risk assessment tools.

1.2.4.2   All individuals assessed as being vulnerable to pressure ulcers should, as a minimum provision, be placed on a high-specification foam mattress with pressure-relieving properties. **B**

1.2.4.3   Although there is no research evidence that high-tech pressure relieving mattresses and overlays are more effective than high-specification (low-tech) foam mattresses and overlays, professional consensus recommends that consideration should be given to the use of alternating pressure or other high-tech pressure-relieving systems: **D**
   ■ as a first-line preventative strategy for people at elevated risk as identified by holistic assessment
   ■ when the individual's previous history of pressure ulcer prevention and/or clinical condition indicates that he or she is best cared for on a high-tech device
   ■ when a low-tech device has failed.

* Since the guideline on pressure ulcer prevention and assessment was published (see Section 5) a study in Australia has suggested that natural sheepskin may be effective in pressure ulcer prevention.

1.2.4.4 All individuals undergoing surgery and assessed as being vulnerable to pressure ulcers should, as a minimum provision, be placed on either a high-specification foam theatre mattress or other pressure-redistributing surface. **D**

1.2.4.5 The provision of pressure-relieving devices needs a 24-hour approach. It should include consideration of all surfaces used by the patient. **D**

1.2.4.6 Support surface and positioning needs should be assessed and reviewed regularly and determined by the results of skin inspection, and patient comfort, ability and general state. Thus repositioning should occur when individuals are on pressure-relieving devices. **D**

GLOSSARY

Abscess   a collection of pus which has localized. It is formed by the liquefactive disintegration of tissue and a large accumulation of polymorphonuclear leucocytes

Albumin   a water-soluble protein. Serum albumin is the chief protein of blood plasma. It is formed principally in the liver and makes up about four-sevenths of the 6–8% protein concentration in the plasma

Alginates   a group of wound dressings derived from seaweed

Anaerobic bacteria   bacteria which thrive in an anoxic environment

Angiogenesis   the process of new blood vessel formation

Antibiotic   a chemical substance that is able to kill or inhibit the growth of micro-organisms. Antibiotics are classified according to their action on the micro-organism

Arteriosclerosis   a group of diseases characterized by thickening and loss of the elasticity of the arterial walls

Aseptic technique   a method of carrying out sterile procedures so that there is the minimum risk of introducing infection. Achieved by the sterility of equipment and a non-touch method

Autolysis   the breakdown of devitalized tissues. The disintegration of cells or tissues by endogenous enzymes

Bacteria   any prokaryotic organism. These are single-celled micro-organisms which lack a true nucleus and organelles. A single loop of double-stranded DNA makes up their genetic material

Callus   localized hyperplasia of the horny layer of the epidermis which is caused by friction or pressure

Cauterization   the application of heat sufficient to scar tissue; used to obtain haemostasis

Cellulitis   inflammation of the subcutaneous tissues. It is characterized by oedema, redness, pain and loss of function

Collagen   the main protein constituent of white fibrous tissue (skin, bone, tendon, cartilage and connective tissue). It is composed of bundles of tropocollagen molecules, which contain three intertwined polypeptide chains

Colonization   the presence of commensal or pathogenic organisms which multiply on the wound but do not cause infection

Contractures	abnormal shortening of muscle or scar tissue rendering the muscle highly resistant to stretching. A contracture can lead to permanent disability
Debridement	the removal of foreign matter or devitalized, injured, infected tissue from a wound until the surrounding healthy tissue is exposed
Dehiscence	a splitting open or separation of the layers of a surgically closed wound
Devitalized	devoid of vitality or life; dead
Doppler ultrasonography	a method of measuring blood flow in peripheral arteries. Changes in blood flow may be correlated with pressure gradients across stenosed vessels and valves and can give an indication of blood supply to the distal tissues
Endothelium	the layer of epithelial cells that line the cavities of the heart and of the blood and lymph vessels and of the serous cavities of the body
Epithelialization	the growth of epithelium over a denuded wound surface
Eschar	dead, devitalized tissue
Extravasation	a discharge or escape of blood or fluid from a vessel in the tissues. Commonly associated with intravenous infusions
Exudate	wound fluid with a high content of protein and cells that has escaped from blood vessels
Fibroblast	an immature collagen-producing cell of connective tissue
Fungate	to produce fungus-like growths; to grow rapidly
Granulation tissue	the new tissue formed during the proliferative phase of wound healing. It consists of connective tissue cells and ingrowing young vessels which form a cicatrix
Haematoma	a localized collection of blood which can form in an organ, space or tissue
Haemostasis	the process of stopping bleeding which can occur naturally by clot formation and artificially by compression or suturing
Hydrocolloid	a dressing material made up of a colloid in which water is the dispersion medium
Hydrogel	a dressing material which consists of a water-containing gel
Hypergranulation/ outgranulation	exuberant amounts of soft, oedematous granulation tissue developing during healing
Hypertrophic	an increase in volume of tissue produced by enlargement of existing cells

Incidence	the proportion of a defined group of patients developing pressure ulcers in a defined period of time
Infection	the invasion and multiplication of micro-organisms in body fluids or tissues. The spectrum of infection agents continually changes as bacteria and viruses are capable of rapid mutation
Inflammation	the initial response to tissue injury. The inflammatory response can be caused by physical, chemical and biological agents
Ischaemia	the deficiency in blood supply to a part of the body due to functional constriction or actual obstruction of a blood vessel
Keloid	a type of scar which is often red and prominent. It is caused by excessive collagen formation in the corium during connective tissue repair
Keratin	an insoluble protein forming the principal component of epidermis, hair, nails and tooth enamel
Leucocytes	the colourless blood corpuscles whose chief function is to protect the body against micro-organisms
Lymphocyte	a mononuclear, non-granular leucocyte, chiefly a product of lymphoid tissue, which participates in the immune response
Maceration	excessive moisture and redness in the tissues surrounding a wound edge
Macrophage	any of the large, mononuclear, phagocytic cells derived from monocytes that are found in the walls of blood vessels and in loose connective tissue. They become stimulated by inflammation on initial angiogenesis
Matrix	the intracellular substance of a tissue which forms the framework of tissues
Maturation	a phase in wound healing where scar tissue is remodelled
Myofibroblast	a differentiated fibroblast containing the ultrastructural features of a fibroblast and a smooth muscle cell and containing many actin-rich microfilaments
Necrosis/ necrotic tissue	the death of previously viable tissue
Prevalence	the proportion of a defined group of patients who already have a pressure ulcer in a defined period of time
Proliferation	the growth or reproduction of tissue as part of the healing process
Proline	a cyclic amino acid occurring in proteins; it is a major constituent of collagen

Pus   a protein-rich liquid which consists of exudate, dead macrophages and bacteria

Scab   the dry crust forming over an open wound which consists of skin and debris

Septicaemia   blood poisoning, a systemic disease where pathogenic micro-organisms are present and multiply in the blood. A life-threatening disease

Slough   a mass of dead tissue in or cast out of living tissue

Suppuration   formation of discharge or pus

Suture   a stitch or series of stitches made to secure opposition of the edges of a surgical or traumatic wound

USEFUL WEBSITE ADDRESSES

General information on wound care

Advances in Skin and Wound Care/Wound Care Communications Network: www.woundcarenet.com

American Academy of Wound Management: www.aawm.org

American Association of Diabetes Educators: www.diabetesnet.com/aade.html

American Burn Association: www.ameriburn.org

American Diabetes Association: www.diabetes.org

American Society of Plastic and Reconstructive Surgery: www.plasticsurgery.org

Australian Wound Management Association: www.awma.com.au

Cochrane Databases: www.update-software.com/clibhome/clib.htm (subscription only)

European Wound Management Association: www.leahcim.demon.co.uk/ewma.htm

http://faculty.uca.edu/glenn.irion/woundelective/adv_wound_management.htm

National Institute for Clinical Excellence (NICE): www.nice.org.uk

National Pressure Ulcer Advisory Panel: www.npuap.org

NHS Centre for Reviews and Dissemination: www.york.ac.uk/inst/crd/welcome.htm

Nursing and Midwifery Council: www.nmc-uk.org

Royal College of Nursing (RCN): www.rcn.org.uk

Society for Vascular Surgery: www.vascsurg.org

Tissue Viability Society: www.tvs.org.uk

World Wide Wounds: www.smtl.co.uk/WMPRC/index.html

Wound Care: www.healthlinksusa.com

Wound Care Information Network: http://medicaledu.com/wndguide.htm

Wound Care Institute: http://woundcare.org/

Wound Care Society: www.woundcaresociety.org

Wounds: a compendium of clinical research and practice: www.woundsresearch.com

www.brpharma.com/woundhealing.htm

www.internurse.com

www.thatnursingsite.com/jcn/abcd

Company sites

Beiersdorf: www.beiersdorf.de/

Clinimed: www.clinimed.co.uk

Coloplast: www.coloplast.com

ConvaTec: www.convatec.com

Hartmann: www.hartmann-online.com

Johnson & Johnson: http://jnj.com

KCI Medical: www.kcimedical.co.uk

3M: www.3m.com

Maersk: www.maersk-medical.com
Molnlycke: www.molnlyckehc.com or www.tendra.com
SSL International: www.seton scholl.com
Smith & Nephew Medical: www.smith-nephew.com

SUBJECT INDEX

Notes: Page numbers followed by 'f' and 't' refer to figures and tables/boxed material respectively.

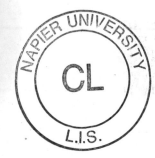